Albert E. Carter's
Rebound Exercise

Contributions & Edits by
Darren Albert Carter,
B.S., R.C.S., Certified Reboundologogist

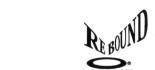

American Institute of Reboundology®

993 N. 450 W.
Springville, Utah 84663
1 (888) 464-JUMP (5867)
www.Rebound-AIR.com

Published by American Institute of Reboundology, Inc. 10/01/2014

ISBN: 978-0-9907972-0-3

This book is printed on acid-free paper.

For more information on rebounding please contact us at:
ReboundAIR, Inc.
993 N. 450 W.
Springville, Utah 84663
1 (888) 464-JUMP (5867)
www.Rebound-AIR.com

Contents

For more information, contact:

www.Rebound-Air.com
Facebook.com/ReboundAir
Toll Free 1-888-464-JUMP

www.GoRebound.com
The Rebound Exercise Documentary

Preface

Rebound exercise just may be the greatest medical discovery since penicillin!

I realize that this statement may be challenged because of the amazing scientific advancements of the last century, but almost all of the medical discoveries are designed to be used to control a pre-existing medical condition. Rebound exercise just happens to be a therapeutic modality that quite possibly eliminates the potential for the medical need for the amazing medications created by our best laboratories.

Albert E. Carter, a non-medical person, has taken the written information of Arthur C. Guyton's Medical Physiology among other great resources and has put it into practical use by presenting it in layman's terms so that anybody can simply understand how the well-being of their own physical body can be improved by participating in a non-invasive, preventative, therapeutic physical activity.

We have known for years that exercise extends and enhances a person's life, but Carter is not satisfied with pat answers. In this book he explains why and how this is true.

The concept of a "cellular exercise" is so simple, refreshing and true. It is a wonder that other fitness experts have not discovered this before.

Understanding the combining effect of the forces of acceleration, deceleration and gravity on the human body is pure genius! This is not to say that nobody else could have done it. It's just that nobody else did.

I rebound daily. And because of the information in this book I know why I rebound daily. I am able to monitor my own physical improvements almost as if I am made of glass and can see each group of cells making their necessary adjustments to the most efficient, effective form of exercise yet devised by man.

Thank you, Albert Carter. Because of you I may not need any of the miracle medications created by our scientists.

Michael D. Riley, M.D.

Chapter One

Finally the Olympics

The word *Olympics* conjures up great dreams of highly qualified and dedicated humans striving for physical perfection in earned talents. The Olympic games bring together thousands of the world's finest athletes to compete against one another. No other sporting event attracts so much attention. Several million people attend the games and hundreds of millions throughout the world watch them on television. Individually, each contestant asks the inner person, "What are my personal physical limits?" Collectively, we spectators ask, "What are our human bodies capable of? How close are we to man's limits? Is there a 'beyond physical limits'? Is it achievable in this life? Will we somehow see it happen on television?"

The Summer Olympics are very special to me.

I was a competitor.

No. You did not see me on television.

My name was not mentioned.

I was not there on the podium, but I was a competitor.

I qualified twice. The first time was in '64 and the second time in '68. My sport was wrestling. My college was Oklahoma State University. I am one of those who will never know what might have been. You see I was eliminated from competition in '64 not by my competitors. I was eliminated because one of my teammates broke my nose and the team doctor would not let me compete. In '68 I separated my rib during practice. I had reached my physical limitations twice.

I consider myself to be among the competitors who are used by the best to become even better. We help make them who they are so, we thrill in their glory. You don't see us on the podium, but we are there.

The Summer Olympics 2000, held in Sydney, Australia were very poignant for me. My wife could not believe I, a grown man, was sitting in my front room in front of the television with tears of emotion streaming down my face. Side glances from my family didn't stop them. And I didn't try to wipe them away. I was seeing history in the making and I did not want to miss a moment of it.

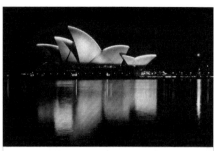

Sydney Opera House, Sydney Australia, Sponsor of the 2000 Summer Olympic Games.

There it was, my other sport, my fetish, my all consuming athletic activity and the object of my profession for over forty-five years. Trampolining was finally introduced and accepted into the Olympics as a sport! And George Nissen, my mentor, the inventor of the trampoline, was honored.

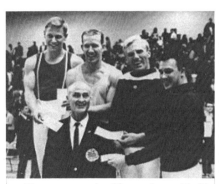

Nissen sponsored and financed many World Professional Trampoline Championships in the late 1960s and early 1970s.

Before the end of his life the trampoline competitors from all over the world paid tribute in front of millions of television spectators.

And rightly so. In 1936, he created a gymnastic device that made it possible for athletes to achieve many different gymnastic moves that had previously been unimaginable and, therefore, unachievable. That very first week of Olympic Trampoline Competition in 2000, we saw double and triple somersaults, double and triple twists and many combinations thereof performed over 35 feet in the air.

Unlike the high divers that perform an intricate dive, splash in the water and receive a score, the trampolinists perform an intricate trampoline move, land on the trampoline and immediately bounce into another intricate move. This happens eight times before they receive their scores.

One of the proudest men during Sydney 2000 must have been 86 year old American George Nissen. Sixty-four years ago, George invented the trampoline and the sport he gave birth to was finally recognized as a full-fledged Olympic event in Sydney. This piece of equipment, which has been responsible for countless banged knees and chipped teeth, first came to Nissen's mind when he worked at the circus as a boy.

Although the elephants were his responsibility, it was the trapeze that fired his imagination. Along with the trapeze was the safety net, but in his imagination, he wanted to be able to land in the net and bounce back up to the trapeze.

"It's been a long journey," says Nissen, whose every public appearance is still graced with a handstand.

It certainly has been a long journey. Early attempts at building his bouncing device involved his bed, some inner tubes and the wrath of his mother.

The Sydney 2000 Olympic trampoline competition was spellbinding. The talent of the participants was beyond belief, but Olympic Trampolining is a brand new event. In the future Olympics, watch for new trampoline moves that have never been performed by man. "That was always my goal and dream," said Nissen. "The struggle and the journey—that's the Olympic spirit."

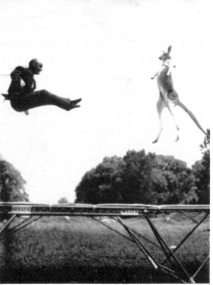

George Nissen jumps with a kangaroo in this 1955 publicity stunt. George would bounce with the kangaroos again in 2000 at the Summer Olympic Games.

Trampoline Competition is not for Everyone

Not every one who has the desire to jump on a trampoline can actually compete. It takes a very special person, one who has been honed to the very finest degree of physical perfection. To be able to achieve the intricate acrobatics, a person has to be able to bounce high enough to allow sufficient airtime to accomplish the desired number of somersaults and twists.

An Olympic high diver achieves his/her altitude by climbing a ladder to the platform. A trampolinist has to create his/her altitude by using the muscles of his/her own legs to bounce. To get high enough, one has to have developed the physique to jump to the necessary altitudes and then be strong enough to handle the landing on the trampoline bed. An Olympic high diver does not need a strong physique to enter the water.

According to NASA, a trampolinist who is jumping thirty-five feet in the air is landing at 8Gs. That is eight times the gravitational pull of the earth. So, a person who weighs 175 pounds on a scale would be hitting the trampoline at 1400 pounds! That is enough to crush the disks and break the bones of an average athlete of other Olympic Events.

While watching an expert trampolinist perform his/her routines one seldom thinks about the affect landing on a trampoline from great heights might have to his/her internal organs. All organs, intestines, stomach, spleen, kidneys, liver, heart and lungs of a human are held in place by connective tissues which are similar to the ligaments and tendons of the musculoskeletal system.

If these connective tissues are weak, the bottom of the bounce could be devastating. The increased weight of each organ could cause it to tear away from the anchoring connective tissues. It would then fall to the bottom of the abdominal cavity. This condition, known as prolapsed organs, is also prevalent among female runners, especially after childbirth. Because the baby and placenta are no longer taking up space in the mother's abdominal cavity, the mother's organs are loose in the abdominal cavity. The trauma of hitting a hard, unforgiving surface with the feet and legs creates such trauma in the abdomen that the uterus and kidneys shear away from their original positions.

Trampolinists run a high risk of prolapsed organs because of the trauma of withstanding up to 8Gs of force with each landing. This means the connective tissues of their bodies also need to be toned and tightened. The trampolinist can only be trained to withstand this type of trauma by training on a trampoline.

The trampolinist also has to be accurate

Each landing has to be achieved so, the trajectory of the competitor's body is as close to vertical as possible. This is because after going thirty-five feet in the air the trampolinist has to be able to land in the middle of the trampoline again, not only for a better score, but also for his or her own safety. A very slight mistake could throw the trampolinist off the trampoline. I know. It has happened to me more than once. The neuromuscular responses of the body simply cannot be miscalculated.

How does the trampolinist achieve such phenomenal physique and balance? It is not possible by lifting weights, swimming, doing calisthenics, yoga, dynamic tension or running on a track. There is only one piece of equipment that the trampolinist can use to help him achieve what he needs—the Olympic trampoline. Trampolining is the only way the vestibular system, the antigravity muscles, the proprioceptors, the brain stem and the nerves in the foot pads can be adequately stimulated to achieve the perfect balance, coordination and timing required by a high flying trampolinist. A trampolinist who finally achieves her competitive edge finds all other exercise methods are ineffective and obsolete.

Perhaps a historical look at how today's exercise systems evolved will help us understand why a trampolinist's method of preparation is different from all other athletes.

Chapter Two

The Genesis of the Olympics

Let us travel to the valley of Olympia to the stadium of Olympia near Athens, Greece and back in time to 350 B.C. to the first known Olympic Games. They were primarily a part of a religious festival in honor of Zeus, the father of the Greek gods and goddesses. The festival and the games were held in a rural sanctuary in the western Peloponnesos in Macedonia.

The stadium could hold 40,000 spectators. Those who attended, all male, watched to see who of all the naked athletes could run the fastest, jump the highest and throw the discus or the javelin the farthest. Hunting

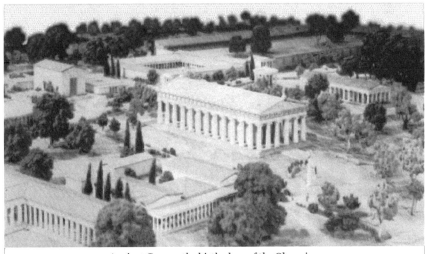

Ancient Greece, the birth place of the Olympics.

skills (the bow and arrow) and fighting skills (javelin, sword, wrestling and boxing) were also displayed.

There were no stopwatches or starting pistols. But most of the time, those who competed and won were those who were prepared by carrying on exercise programs designed by their personal coaches. The coaches knew if certain things happened to the athlete's muscles, they would get stronger. If the athletes ran for long distances during practice, they would be able to run longer in competition. They knew that because they trained horses this way.

As athletic competition spread across the civilized world, so also did the need for coaches and athletic instructors. They studied the human body to determine how to make it faster, stronger, harder and able to endure longer.

The coaches, many times family members, understood how the muscles worked by making comparisons to wild game and other animals they killed and slaughtered. As they would pull the skin off of a deer, they would see how the muscles were connected to the bones by tendons. By experimentation with athletes, coaches soon found certain actions done under tension would cause a group of muscles to become stronger.

It was not too long before coaches were creating devices that would cause the muscles to strain under different loads. Possibly pulling wagons or sleds was a method of stimulating the muscles of the legs to become stronger. Clearing land by lifting rocks onto the wagons, I am sure, was also used.

It doesn't take too much of an imagination to realize that the coaches who wanted to make names for themselves soon created a work yard where the athletes would come and lift and carry heavy wagon wheels, axles, rocks, iron bars and other weights. And I imagine it took only one rainstorm to force the athletes to pick up all of the weights they could carry and run or waddle into the closest barn. And thus the first weight lifting club was created.

Men are enterprising. With the demand of creating competitive athletes, more weight lifting establishments sprang up in every community. Foundries began to create calibrated weights and bars to sell to the weight lifting clubs. The weight lifting clubs began to compete with each other. Other exercise devices using benches, pulleys, levers, arms, ropes and cables began to show up. The sales representative who sold each created device to the weight lifting clubs explained how and why his new device was better for a very specific group of muscles.

Weight training stations were established. Then the athletes were informed that if they wanted to have the perfect body they would have to spend time at each weight lifting station.

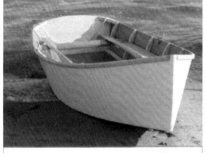
Predecessor to the rowing machine.

I don't know when the running tracks were added. It is possible they were always there in the form of a dusty road or a trail through the woods. But I am sure each athlete was told that when they finished their weight lifting they had to do their roadwork.

When the bicycle was invented, rather than running, some of the athletes preferred riding the bicycle. Then when a bicycle broke down or inclement weather set in or both, the stationary bicycle was invented.

It doesn't take too much imagination to figure where the rowing machine came from.

But it's the treadmill that takes some explanation. As scientists began to study the human body and the effect running had on it, they needed to somehow connect electrical monitors to various parts of the body so, they could record the action of the lungs and the heart. Because the electronic monitoring device was stationary and the wires were short, the scientists needed to keep the subject's body in a comparatively stationary location. The treadmill was created for that purpose. But just as the stationary bicycle found its way into the weight training clubs, so also did the treadmill.

Not much has changed. Oh, the dead weights are more calibrated. The weight training stations are chromed, adjustable and more user friendly.

Mirrors, carpets, televisions, drinking fountains, fruit bars, saunas and hot tubs have been added. The coaches are still the same. They still teach the same thing. Mentally they dissect the body by groups of muscles and present a specific exercise for each part of the body. The new and improved exercise devices still stimulate only the specific group of muscles for which it was made. You need to go to several exercise stations to exercise all of your skeletal muscles and when finished you need your road work, either on a running track, a stationary bicycle or an elliptical machine.

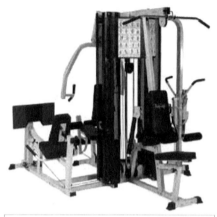

Home gym designed to work specific muscle groups one at a time.

Today's Health Clubs are Lacking

Believe it or not, today's health clubs do not claim to exercise the entire body. Although exercise does strengthen the bones, the health experts do not hold classes for the purpose of strengthening the skeleton. The involuntary muscles of digestion and elimination are overlooked as if they are not part of the body. The eyes and inner ears, used for balance, are also overlooked. Even the lymphatic system is denied existence in a health club.

In the same period of time exercise has evolved to what it is, transportation has changed from walking, running, riding horses and buggies to automobiles, airplanes and SUVs. Communication has changed from yelling across the field to using cell phones and the Internet.

There is no denying the methods used in today's exercise establishments do work. The experts have had literally thousands of years to perfect them and teach them to their students. One cannot argue with thousands of universities who have athletes who are training under the tutorship of athletic trainers and coaches. After all, haven't the athletic trainers and coaches been trained by their trainers and coaches? They know what they are doing. Besides it costs hundreds of thousands of dollars to equip the modern weight training facility that services the university and athletic teams. Well, if it isn't broke, don't fix it.

Still, there is something wrong with conventional exercise. There are no normal stresses which the body is exposed to that even nearly approach

the extreme stresses of heavy exercise. In fact, if some of the extremes
of exercise were continued for even
slightly prolonged periods of time,
the results might easily be lethal.

When a person who has an extremely high fever, approaching a
lethal level, the body's metabolism
increases to about 100% above normal. Compare that to the metabolism
of the body during a marathon race
when the metabolism is elevated
nearly 2000% above normal.

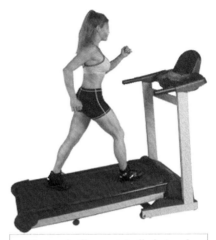

The final common denominator
in athletic events is what the muscles
can do for you, what strength they

The treadmill was originally designed so
that scientists and healthcare professionals
could measure the effects of running on the
body.

can give when it is needed, what power they can achieve in the performance
of work and how long they can continue in their activity.

The strength of a muscle is determined mainly by its size. A maximum
contractile force is between 2.5 kg and 3.5 kg per cm^2 of muscle cross-sectional area. Thus, a man who has enlarged muscles will be much stronger
than a man without that advantage. So, the athlete who has hypertrophied
his or her muscles through exercise likewise will have increased muscle
strength because of increased muscle size.

To give an example of muscle strength, a world-class weight lifter
might have a quadriceps muscle with a cross-sectional area as great as 150
cm^2. This would translate into a maximum contractile strength of 525 kg
(or 1155 lb). All this force is applied to the patellar tendon. Therefore, one
can readily understand how it is possible for this tendon to be ruptured
even avulsed from its insertion into the tibia below the knee. Also, when
such tension is exerted on tendons that span a joint, similar forces are also
applied to the surfaces of the joints or sometimes to ligaments spanning the
joints. This accounts for such happenings as displaced cartilages, compression fractures around the joint and torn ligaments.

To make matters still worse, the holding strength of muscles is about
40 percent greater than the contractile strength. So, if a muscle is already
contracted and a force then attempts to stretch out the muscle, this
requires about 40 per cent more force than is required by a shortening
contraction. Therefore, the above mentioned 525 kg of force on the patel-

lar tendon becomes 735 kg (1617 lb). This added stress obviously com-pounds the problems of the tendons, joints and ligaments. It can also lead to internal tearing in the muscle itself. In fact, stretching a maximally contracted muscle is one of the best ways to insure the highest degree of muscle soreness.

Is it possible the old fashioned weight training and road work concept of body building may be hazardous to your health?

Chapter Three

The Search

A trampolinist is writing this book. So, its views and conclusions are obviously very biased. Some people have dreams of flying. I didn't. As a child I had a reoccurring disconcerting dream that would come to me sometimes twice a week. I would dream the entire world was made of green JELL-O®. In my dreams, instead of walking, I would bounce. At first I would bounce over fences, then houses and trees. I would always come down and if I didn't land in a tree or on a house, I knew the ground would be soft and bouncy and it would catapult me into the air again. They were fun dreams.

"Carter, get off that trampoline!"

I can still hear coach Bill Stalling's voice ring across the gymnasium as he came in and caught me bouncing on the Columbia Falls High School trampoline again. He didn't mind my bouncing; he just didn't want me using the trampoline when the girls were supposed to be using it.

It was only a few minutes previous to Stallings' chastisement that I had received permission from him to be excused from my freshman study hall to go to the gym and help instruct the girls on how to bounce. It was obvious the coach wanted me to instruct, not demonstrate. It's just that I couldn't stay away from the trampoline. I was addicted to the ability of freeing myself from gravity if only for a few seconds.

Ben Yagoda, executive editor of *New Jersey Monthly,* presented an interesting point of view about jumping.

"Along with running, the jump is probably the athletic activity most elemental to human experience. Consider the expression 'jump for joy,' or watch a child as he or she is introduced to a pogo stick or a trampoline and you'll see what I mean."

But what is jumping? In terms of physics, it is one of the most basic expressions of Newton's law of action and reaction. Pushing down against the immovable ground causes the equal and opposite reaction of being propelled into the air. The power of the jump, according to the science of biomechanics (the science of applying the principles of physics to human movement) is called vertical reaction force (VRF).

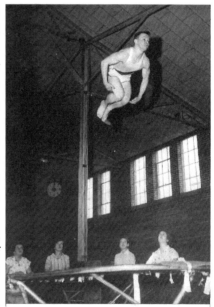

Al Carter begins a triple back somersault on a trampoline.

This is expressed in formula form as $W + ma_y$ where W is the force of gravity on the jumper, m is the body weight (a constant) and a_y is the acceleration.

Important as jumping is to a variety of sports; it is a remarkably good exercise in its own right. That's not so surprising when one considers that it may be the purest of athletic endeavors, a simple contest between the jumper and gravity. This fact was recognized back in 1921 by Dr. Dudley Sargent, who wrote,

"I want to share what seems to me the simplest and most effective of all tests of physical ability with the other fools who are looking for one."

He then introduced the standing high jump. Apparently this was seen to make sense for the Sargent Vertical Jump, in which you mark the highest point you can reach and then see how much higher you can reach by jumping, is still a test of strength widely administered in American schools. Whatever Ben Yagoda and Dr. Sargent discovered about jumping is enhanced dramatically when applied to a trampoline.

I want to speak for the Carter family as we look back at the many rich experiences we have had as a direct result of our knowledge of and involvement in rebound exercise. Daily we are able to compare vital information we have learned from the basic concepts of rebound exercise and confirm information we have been taught by our professors and coaches. Even if that was the only benefit we received from rebound exercise, we are truly blessed.

But there is more I didn't understand about what was happening to me as I bounced on the school trampoline through high school in Columbia Falls, Montana. Still, the extra balance, coordination, strength and stamina developed because of my trampolining made it possible for me to attend Oklahoma State University on a full scholarship for wrestling.

My father moved our family from Montana to Tulsa, Oklahoma to take over the Presidency of the Admiral State Bank between my junior and senior years in high school.

In Tulsa, my peers and fellow wrestlers knew me as the "Montana Hick." This not-so-kind nickname became mine because I was from Montana and because Goodyear Rubber was on strike and I was unable to buy wrestling shoes for the first part of the wrestling year. But when they found I didn't lose wrestling matches, they dropped the "Hick" part from my nickname, "Montana". In my senior year I won the Oklahoma State High School Wrestling Championship, 137 pound weight class for Will Rogers High School.

One day after school in the wrestling room, while waiting to begin wrestling practice, we wrestlers were playing a card game. The stakes were push-ups. It was good that I was better at wrestling than playing cards because at the end of the session I was two hundred push-ups in debt and the other wrestlers wanted me to pay up.

After doing some serious negotiating, they agreed a one armed push-up was equivalent to two two-arm push-ups. At that time I discovered that I could do one hundred one-armed push-ups without stopping!

I paid my debt to the amazement of my fellow wrestlers and myself and gained a great deal of respect. I never played cards for push-ups again, but for the next forty years I did my one hundred one-arm push-ups on my birthday just to prove I could still do them. I don't believe I ever did tie my strong physique in high school and college to my continual trampolining, I simply accepted my strength and agility as God given.

It wasn't until years later that I found out otherwise. My son, Darren, came home from the first grade in Edmonds, Washington bragging, "I did fifteen sit-ups in P. E. today."

"That's great son," I exclaimed proudly, "Were you tired?"

"No."

"Do you think you could do more than fifteen sit-ups?"

"Probably," he said matter-of-factly.

"I want to see how many sit-ups you can do," I challenged. I held his ankles down and began to count as he did his sit-ups."

"... 25, 26, 27," I counted, ".... 150, 151, 152," I continued, "... 300, 301, 302."

"...400, 401, 402," I declared with amazement. I thought he was broken! Who ever heard of any first grader doing that many sit-ups? He finally stopped at 429 sit-ups!

I couldn't believe it. Neither could Wendie, my nine year old daughter who was witnessing this physical feat. But she wasn't about to let her little brother beat her in anything, so, I held her ankles down while she did sit-ups. She stopped at 476 sit-ups, not because she was tired. She stopped because she beat her brother!

Later that year she came home and announced that she humiliated all of the sixth grade boys in arm wrestling even though to my knowledge she had never competed in arm wrestling in her life.

Somehow my children and I were amazingly strong without consciously working for it. Even though our lifestyle was fun and playful, physiologically trampolining and gymnastics was "work" and we benefited from it.

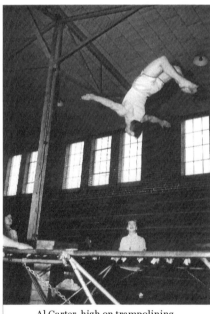

Al Carter, high on trampolining.

That seemed to go against everything I had ever been taught in college. Exercise was supposed to be hard, sweaty and painful. Still, there had to be an answer. What was the common denominator responsible for our family strength? Was it possible to inherit physical strength? Or is physical strength a product of lifestyle? This was worthy of research.

My children and I are products of rebound exercise. I started bouncing on a trampoline at fourteen. I won three state championships as an amateur trampolinist and three State Wrestling Championships. I have performed as a professional trampolinist for the last 35 years.

My Gymnastics Fantastics professional trampoline team toured the U.S. in the 1974–1975, school year under the sponsorship of the Marriott

Corporation. We traveled the United States in our specially-equipped motor home and performed for over half a million people during that year. The Gymnastics Fantastics trampoline team consisted of five year old Darren Carter, (my son and, presently, our company webmaster), eight year old Wendie, (my daughter) and thirty-five year old Dad (yours truly). The Gymnastics Fantastics performed as many as three shows a day five days a week—five hundred trampoline shows in that year.

In 1977, I was introduced to the small round indoor exercise device that looked like a trampoline, except the six legs were only six inches long. The black mat was supported by thirty-six springs. The sales representative tried to tell me it was good for jogging indoors.

"You don't even know what you are talking about," I remember blurting out. "You've got the most efficient, effective form of exercise yet devised by man! I'm a professional trampolinist. I ought to know."

That evening I tried to tell the sales representative why trampolining was so good for the body. I didn't think I did a very good job, but I guess he did because he asked me if I would endorse the use of this funny looking "springy thingy."

Knowing the health benefits I personally received from trampolining and the apparent benefits my children had received, I jumped at the chance. However, I was not willing to write an article without plenty of back up. So, the next day, I was in the library to check out books on health, physiology, human anatomy, aerobics and various exercises.

Among them were books on trampolining, jogging, jumping rope and texts on physical education. My concern, that day, was locating textbooks I could quote. I fully expected to find all the information about what happens to the body while on the trampoline. After all, hadn't I received this information from my trusted gymnastics instructors? And where had they received their information?

That evening, after the children were in bed, I began to study the stack of books on top of the desk in front of me.

Among the books was *Physiology of Exercise*. I was immediately impressed with the author's approach to the subject of exercise and its effect on the health of the human body.

On pages 220 and 221, I found activities listed according to the number of calories burned per hour. The list started with sleeping and ended with horizontal running at 18.9 miles per hour.

Imagine my disappointment when I found trampolining was not among the exercises. Surely, this must be an oversight by the authors.

Anyone who has ever been on a trampoline knows how tired and winded one gets while bouncing. I mean it's not an unknown. Trampolines were available to our elementary, junior high, high school and college students. At one time we had NCAA competitions; and even today we have national and world trampoline competitions.

Trampolining is now an Olympic event. It became so in the Australian 2000 Olympic Games. I concluded that what I needed in order to write about beneficial bouncing was a physiology book with a larger list of exercises so, I made another trip back to the library.

Ah ha. It appeared the library had just what I was looking for. I checked out *The International Guide to Fitness and Health*. Now there's a physiology book! On the front cover it boasted it was, "from the latest research of the International Committee on Standardization, which includes the fields of medicine, nutrition and physical education ... the most authoritative techniques for planning a really workable, enjoyable, individual exercise program."

Surely this book would have just what I was looking for. I found their activities list beginning on page 50 and it continued for five pages! The exercises were in alphabetical order beginning with archery and ending with number 133, yard work. It included such activities as kite flying, putting practice, jai alai, wrestling, tumbling and even piloting a plane. But something was missing. Under the T's, I found no mention of trampolining!

Now, I wasn't just disappointed. I was hurt. If I were a baseball player, my sport would be listed. But I was a trampolinist and mine wasn't there.

For the next two weeks, I searched every library I could find for any physiology books that men-

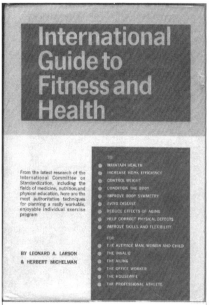

This book, like many other books presenting research on exercise in 1977, totally ignored the benefits of rebounding or trampolining.

tioned trampolining. I found none. I also pulled out all the books I could find on trampolining written by trampolinists, but to my amazement, even these books made no mention of what actually happens to the body while doing tricks.

In desperation, I finally called the Nissen Corporation in Cedar Rapids, Iowa. Surely they could lead me to the proper resources. After all, according to the *Guinness Book of Records*, it was George Nissen who invented the trampoline in 1936. And it was the Nissen equipment I had been working on for the past twenty years. My call went straight through to the top and I talked at some length to Bob Bevenour, Executive Vice President. But to my dismay, I learned he faced the same problem. He said he would like to find any study that explained why trampolining was so good physically. He agreed to send me anything they had in their files that had anything to do with the benefits of bouncing on a trampoline, if I would reciprocate by sending directly to him any found information.

Well, Nissen has been the leader in the trampoline industry for years. If it doesn't have any information on the exercise benefits of trampolining, then I must have been fooling myself all these years. Maybe trampolining was not a better exercise than running, but deep inside I knew it had to be at least as good.

Discouraged, I decided to write a short page about how running on an "indoor jogger" as it was called, was a good alternative to outside running. After all, I guess it was rather self-centered of me to imagine my form of exercise was better than any other exercise.

I was practically sleepless the next week, as I began to return the books to the libraries. Then I asked myself, "Since trampolining was not included in the lists along with all of the other activities, where would it fit in?"

Chapter Four

The Discovery: It's Easy to Fall Down, You Have to Work to Get Up

Gravity, the Common Denominator of All Exercises

Rather than returning the last few books, I sat down at a table in the library and began to thumb through the books looking for the answer that didn't seem to be there. I still had an hour before the library closed. I pulled out a piece of paper and began to write down everything all exercises have in common. Halfway through the list, I stopped. I noticed something in common that I had not noticed before. I scanned the rest of the exercises. I suddenly felt an "ah ha"! It was as if someone had turned on a light inside my brain.

"That's it!" I exclaimed out loud. I stood up and began to pace around the table, my mind moving a million miles a second trying to recall everything I had read in the last couple of weeks.

"It's so simple!" I blurted out loud, "Why haven't I seen this before?"

"Please, Sir. You are disturbing others," the librarian said approaching me.

"All exercises have one thing in common!" I exclaimed to her. "They are all related to gravity."

"That may be sir, but we don't exercise in the library. Please be quiet or I'll have to ask you to leave," she said in a not too hushed voice.

"No." I turned abruptly, walking away from the librarian. "Not just related, they *oppose* the gravitational pull of the earth." I suddenly turned and faced her. " That's it!"

"Sir, are you checking these books in or out?"

"In. No. Out. I have them checked out. I was going to check them in, but now I don't want to. I'll keep them. So, I guess neither."

I abruptly left her stammering and walked out muttering to myself, *"The common denominator of all exercises is the opposition to the gravitational pull of the earth!"*

In front of the library, I sat down in the middle of the sidewalk and opened the books and went over the exercises one at a time to see if it checked.

"What about push-ups? Yes, we are pushing away from gravity. Chin-ups? Of course! We pull the whole body up, up and away from gravity. And sit-ups? Gravity is pulling on our torso as we pull away from the floor. Leg-lifts? We are opposing gravity when our abdominal muscles lift our legs off the floor. What about weight lifting? Sure. The word, "weight" by definition is "mass times gravity."

I stood and began walking away from my pile of books and papers.

"Even the aerobic exercises fit into the category. To walk, (I slowly began walking) you first move your center of gravity in the direction you wish to go until you start falling that direction and then you take a series of steps to keep from falling. Jogging and running (I began methodically jogging) are accomplished by allowing gravity to pull down on the upper body long before taking steps to recover. Walking, jogging and running are simply states of continuous falling, not quite catching your balance until you decide to stop.

"Dancing is falling in various directions," I was beginning to draw a crowd, "while overcompensating with precise steps to change direction and control the rhythm of the fall and recovery.

"Even swimming is directly influenced by the gravitational pull of the earth," I yelled to the curious. "Although the body appears to be defying the law of gravity by floating, floating is not an exercise. Swimming is." I explained to several. "The downward pull of gravity on the water keeps the water in the pool, lake or river. The resistance created by the density of the water molecules make swimming a good exercise for the muscles of the swimmer. Gravity pulls down on the water hard enough to make it dense enough to have something to resist. That resistance is what makes swimming a good exercise."

I came back to my spread of books and my senses at the same time. Every exercise listed was functional as an exercise because it demanded energy to oppose gravity. Trampolining fit and because it did, it deserved the research and acknowledgement that it was an exercise. Just how good? I didn't know, but I was going to find out even if it took me the rest of my life.

I was down—depressed—and then I was up—enthused. I rebounded. It felt good.

Gravity is a Universal Law

Flying across the United States at 37,000 feet, in a very comfortable, climate controlled, pressurized modern Boeing 767 jet plane, I became acutely aware of an interesting fact of my existence. I couldn't see the earth in the darkness of the night and for the moment, the only thing that existed was the pod in which a few fellow human beings were casually eating, snoozing, reading and chatting with one another. But the same physical force we contend with while we are standing on the earth influenced our every move.

The theory of universal gravitation explains that the same force holding the earth in orbit around the sun was also present in the aircraft. That theory states every element in the universe is subject to the effects of gravity from some celestial body. The moon's gravity pulls on the earth and the earth's gravity pulls on the moon. This is evidenced by the moon's influence on the tides as it orbits the earth. Likewise, the liquid in my glass at 37,000 feet pulls as hard on the earth as the earth pulls on the contents of my glass.

Now, we live on the earth. Because of that fact, every one of our bodies is affected dozens of ways by the earth's gravitational pull. How many ways we just don't know.

There are those scientists who believe various species of animals, a large variety of plants, bats and birds and even a great many people are influenced by the moon's gravity. That may be so, but be that as it may, we know gravity is a universal unbreakable law.

In his investigation, Sir Isaac Newton found the strength of gravity depends on two things:

1.   the amount of matter each body contains and
2.   the distance between the bodies.

With this information, Sir Isaac Newton worked out a formula for the strength of gravity between two bodies—any two bodies in the universe. I wonder, if this is where they get the idea of a magnetic personality?

$$F = \frac{M_1 \times M_2}{R_2}$$

In this equation, if F stands for the force of gravity and the amount of matter in one body is M_1; while the amount of matter in the other body is M_2, then R is the distance between the bodies.

When distance = 1 $\qquad F = \dfrac{M_1 \times M_2}{1 \times 1} = \dfrac{1}{1}$

When distance = 2 $\qquad F = \dfrac{M_1 \times M_2}{2 \times 2} = \dfrac{1}{4}$

When distance = 3 $\qquad F = \dfrac{M_1 \times M_2}{3 \times 3} = \dfrac{1}{9}$

In other words, if the mass of the two bodies remains the same, as the distance doubles, the gravitational pull will be reduced by three-fourths. If the distance between them triples, the gravitational pull will be reduced by eight-ninths.

On the earth, two other things determine the strength of the gravitational pull:

The distance of an object from the center of the earth; and the spin of the earth.

For our purposes, although this difference is measurable, it is not important. What is important is that gravity is pulling down on all parts of our body. And since we are subjected to the gravitational pull of the earth, in order to move across the face of the earth, we have to oppose it.

The reason the earth has an atmosphere is because the particles of the air are captured by the earth's gravity.

The device used to measure atmospheric pressure is a barometer, which means, "weight meter." The kind we are most familiar with is a vacuum tube inserted into a dish filled with mercury. The weight of the atmosphere on the outside presses down on the mercury, pushing a column of mercury into the tube. At sea level, the pressure of the atmosphere causes

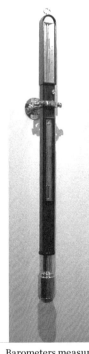

Barometers measure atmospheric pressure.

the mercury column to rise to almost 30 inches. At five thousand feet above sea level, the atmosphere is only able to support a mercury column about 25 inches high.

Changing altitude, whether in a car or an airplane, causes us to swallow several times in order to change the pressure in the inner ear and sinuses. But what we may not realize is gravity has an even greater affect on us because our bodies are made up primarily of liquid and solid structures that react directly to the gravitation of the earth. *So, gravity directly or indirectly influences every cell throughout the entire body.*

Each living cell has the amazing capacity to adjust to the gravitational pull it experiences on earth.

In fact, Gravity is the most important and constant force of our physical existence. Gravity is one of those laws that was decreed in the Heavens before the foundation of the earth was laid. When we learn to understand and use this law, blessings of health, wisdom and great knowledge are ours for the asking.

Opposition is Necessary to Develop Strength

Now, for all intents and purposes, although gravity is pulling down on everything equally, it has a different effect on living things than on dead or inanimate objects, like buildings, rocks, dirt and fallen leaves. On dead or inanimate things, gravity simply pulls them to their final resting place as close to the center of the earth as possible. But on anything that lives, it provides a force that, by necessity, has to be opposed.

You see, one of the differences between dead things and living things is that living things have the ability to follow another law just as important and everlasting as gravity.

What law? Simply stated, *there must be opposition in all things to develop strength.* Dead things cannot develop strength. All living things can and do.

One of the characteristics of all living organisms is their ability to react to changes in their environment. This is true for plants, animals, bacteria, human cells and, of course, human beings.

Giant trees of the Redwood Forest in California grow strong, tall and vertical by opposing gravity. Wheat stalks are given the vertical direction to grow by gravity. The straw stalks oppose gravity. Engineers use plumb bobs, a weight on the end of a string, to determine what is perpendicular to gravity. This ensures that walls and doorframes are built to their strongest.

We are not immune to this ever downward pull. We oppose gravity every day as we move about on the face of the earth.

A newborn baby's first challenge is to lift his arms and legs and eventually his head away from the force that is constantly pulling him down. Gravity, by opposition, becomes the first coach who teaches the baby to crawl, walk, run, jump and play. If these actions are not done correctly, Coach Gravity immediately pulls the

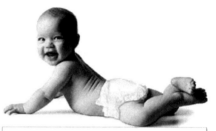

From the very beginning of their lives, babies gain strength by opposing gravity.

infant down to try again. This learning process takes less than a day for a colt or a baby giraffe and years for a human baby.

A child starts life with a basic ability to move with a set of distinguishable movement characteristics. These movements are developed during the first three years of life and specifically refer to the gravitational forces acting upon the body. Against constant opposition, the child stands up and eventually becomes an upright citizen.

Man's upright posture governs the way he experiences the world. The vertical and horizontal axes of perceived space are established only with reference to gravity. His visual clues, identifying vertical, horizontal or diagonal lines only assist the postural ones. The way man sees his world depends on his upright posture. This makes it crucial to maintain correct equilibrium against the pull of gravity. For man to function properly, he must be in harmony with earth's gravitational pull.

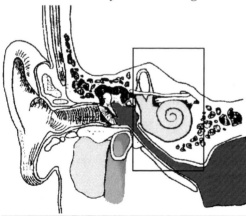

The inner ear has as much to do with equilibrium and balance as it has to do with hearing.

Our amazing bodies are designed to achieve equilibrium automatically after the basics in movement and balance are learned. Small sensory hairs in the inner ear are affected by the relationship between gravity and the position. The semicircular ducts in the inner ear are the sense organs of dynamic equilibrium. They are responsible for making sure the head is at a right angle to the horizontal plane of the earth. This is what is known as the head righting reflex.

To coordinate body position, there are nerve receptors in the feet and the rest of the body that relay to the brain stem the relationship of the body to the gravitational force. Impulses from these widely located sensory receptors integrate and converge on a final pathway to bring about effective and coordinated responses of the antigravity muscles.

Strengthening these muscles by proper vigorous exercise helps us to retain or recover normal orientation in space. Equilibrium occurs when we can identify exactly where we are relative to the gravitational pull of the earth.

The free movements of a ballet dancer, a gymnast, a trampolinist or any other athlete attempt to obtain freedom of movement through exercise. This symbolizes man's aspiration to advance, to rise farther above the earth, to challenge, to live, to achieve and to oppose the downward pull of gravity. When these are achieved, the student has learned his or her lessons well, all taught by Coach Gravity.

Some people feel that constantly opposing gravity for an entire life is too much to ask. They decide to simply give in, to surrender to this constant urge. Their constrictive movements symbolize fatigue, withdrawal, defeat and resignation. A catatonic patient may assume the fetal position. This is an example of the living refusing to live, refusing to oppose gravity and finally accepting death.

Chapter Five

Albert Einstein's Surprising Contribution to the Ideal Exercise

During the next few weeks I spent every spare moment, and even some I couldn't spare, writing and rewriting the manuscript of *Rebound to Better Health*. The book began to take shape; the arguments were labored, but convincing. However, there was still something missing. I knew there had to be something more than just opposing gravity, but I couldn't quite put my fingers on it. Finally, after several nights of writing and rewriting, I came to a fatigued and dismal halt.

That night, after midnight, I was alone at my desk. I felt trapped by my commitment and not able to do anything about it.

"Oh God, what am I not seeing?" I prayed. I got up from my desk and went to a set of encyclopedias, *The New Book of Knowledge,* and looked up "gravity" on page 320 in volume 7. Gloom descended as I read: "For 300 years scientists have studied gravitation. They can measure its strength and tell other things about it, but the question, 'What is gravitation?' is still a mystery."

I continued to read:

"In 1911, the famous scientist, Albert Einstein, developed a new idea of gravitation. He showed that gravitation and acceleration produced the same effects. There is no way [for the human body] to tell gravitation from acceleration or deceleration."

I looked up from the book in a half daze. "That's it!" I said aloud. "That's what's missing! I've found it!"

I leaped from my chair, grabbed the book and tripped up the stairs to our bedroom where my wife lay sleeping.

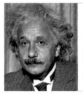

Albert Einstein's discovery about gravity led to amazing discoveries about rebounding.

"I found the key! I found what I've been looking for and it's been in the basement all the time!"

"You found what?" she asked, trying to wake up.

"The key," I exclaimed, out of breath.

"I didn't know we had lost one."

"Listen, when we jump there is more than one force we are working with!"

"Let's talk about it in the morning," she said, rolling over and pulling the covers over her head.

"How can you sleep when I'm so excited?"

"I can't. So, I'll listen," she said, sitting up. "Now, you said you found a missing key in our basement?"

"The answer explaining why bouncing or rebounding is as good as or better than all other exercises! We've been talking about opposing gravity. All exercises do that, but acceleration is a completely different force. Although it's different, the human body can't tell the difference. Therefore, if you accelerate vertically like in a rocket ship or on a trampoline, you develop a greater G-Force."

"Oh, I get it," she brightened, "If you come down and stop, you decelerate and for just a moment the body feels the combined effects of deceleration and gravity and responds like somebody had suddenly turned up the earth's gravitational pull."

"Right. Albert Einstein explains that acceleration comes in two types. Acceleration is the change in velocity of matter. Either it is increasing in velocity or decreasing in velocity. It is either positive or negative velocity."

"Well, to the average person this positive and negative velocity is known as acceleration and deceleration."

"Right. And where do these forces come together for just a moment?"

"At the bottom of the bounce?" she asked, timidly.

"Exactly. That might explain why I can still do over one hundred one arm push-ups although I have never lifted weights. Is it possible that my entire body has adjusted to a greater G-Force environment. Is it because I am a trampolinist?"

"If that's the case, all trampolinists should have extra unexplained physical strength."

"Right. Who do we know who are trampolinists?"

"Our children. Both Darren and Wendie have been on the trampoline since before they could walk."

"And that is why they are much stronger without even trying."

For the next two hours, we brainstormed and things began to fall into place. The next day, I researched Arthur C. Guyton's *Medical Physiology*, The chapter entitled "Space Physiology" verified what we had discovered. There it was. The federal government had already spent millions investigating the effects of acceleration and deceleration on our astronauts both horizontally and vertically. However, those studies were designed to see how much G-Force the body could stand without physical damage or blacking out, not how much was needed to enhance the health or strength of the physical body.

One thing is sure. The force of acceleration (both positive and negative) does exist. And we don't even have to pay for it. It is ours for FREE. So, let's take a closer look at acceleration.

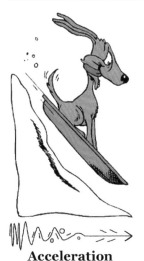

Acceleration

Acceleration—Overlooked, but powerful

It is amazing how we are able to travel today. In the days of King Solomon the royal method of travel was on the back of a donkey or possibly in a wagon or chariot. But when we want to go to another location, we hop in an automobile and step on the gas or the accelerator. The increasing speed of the forward motion of the automobile pushes us back into the seat. We feel the force of acceleration. With all of his wisdom, it is possible King Solomon never experienced the force of acceleration.

In the late forties and early fifties test pilots were strapped into jet sleds that ran across the desert on smooth rails. The sleds were allowed to accelerate so fast the men experienced G-Forces nine or ten times that of gravity. This was necessary to find out if the future astronauts would be able to withstand the seven G-Force expected during liftoff. That increased G-Force meant a 175 pound astronaut would weigh 1,225 pounds immediately after liftoff. All cells individually would be seven times heavier. Would cell membranes be able to withstand the increased G-Force or would the cells rupture and die?

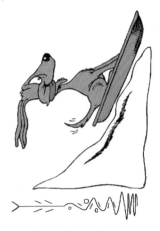

Deceleration

Deceleration—Yet Another Force?

If in a moving automobile, it becomes desirable to slow down or stop, we apply the brakes or the decelerator. We experience a force known as negative acceleration. We commonly call it deceleration. We use deceleration all the time. A carpenter, using a hammer, drives a nail with the force of deceleration or negative acceleration. The acceleration of the head of the hammer is expended against the head of the nail.

During early space flight when the astronauts returned to earth, they experienced another increase in their body weight during the negative acceleration or the deceleration part of their re-entry flight. The huge drag parachutes opened to slow the landing module during reentry into the earth's atmosphere and the astronaut's bodies increased in weight by at least 4.5Gs. One of the G-Forces was the earth's gravity, but the other 3.5Gs were identified as 3.5Gs of deceleration. However, the cells of their bodies accepted this change as an increase in gravity and, no doubt, acted accordingly.

I felt the force of acceleration when my Boeing jet began to increase to flight speed as it rolled down the runway for take off. Although I was trying to lean forward to look out the window, the acceleration force pushed me back into my seat. After the flight when the plane touched down, my body strained against the seat belt until we had slowed sufficiently to turn and taxi to our gate.

It is hard for me to comprehend that although our space scientists have studied the effects of these forces on our bodies, they haven't used this information to develop a space age exercise. Sometimes the simplicity of an idea completely mystifies our scientists, but is easily understood by the common man. I was explaining the rebound concept to an audience in Pennsylvania when a bearded Amish gentleman stood up. He said,

"Mr. Carter, what you are trying to tell us is that it appears we have three natural forces available to us at no cost that we should use to exercise effectively, but we haven't been harnessing them up right."

"What do you mean?" I asked.

"Well, if I had three powerful horses hooked up to one plow with one pulling to the right, one pulling to the left and one pulling straight ahead, I would have a hard time plowing my field, wouldn't I?"

"You have the idea exactly," I said. We have accepted the forces of acceleration and deceleration as parts of our environment because they exist, but we haven't considered even for a moment the combined therapeutic impact of these forces on the human body. We know they exist. We know everybody has to cope with them. But what's the most efficient way to use them? Obviously, our Amish farmer will get more plowing done by making sure all three horses pull in the same direction. So, by lining up the effects of acceleration and deceleration with gravity, it stands to reason that these forces will have a greater impact on our bodies.

Oh, that's just too simple!

The Vertical Stacking of Natural Forces— Just for the Health of it

The gravitational force pulling on everything on this earth is vertical. As long as we live here on Mother Earth, we are subject to gravity. Although we are constantly affected by it, we cannot control it or change it. However, we can control the direction and intensity of the forces of acceleration and deceleration.

A baseball pitcher depends upon his or her ability to accelerate the baseball to between seventy and a hundred miles an hour towards the home plate. A batter's objective is to accelerate the bat in the opposite direction so the ball decelerates to a complete stop. Then he or she must accelerate it in the opposite direction to a speed that will carry the ball out of the ballpark. This speed needs to be achieved before the atmospheric friction slows the ball down enough for gravity to capture it. When the batter fails, a catcher uses his or her glove to decelerate the ball.

Although these forces have been in existence ever since mass was acted upon by force, we have never considered them as viable tools when it comes to exercising the body. Gravity has been used forever, but these other two forces have been overlooked. They are not talked about in the health clubs or the training rooms. They are not published. They are not presented in physical education classes in high schools or colleges. Perhaps the reason acceleration and deceleration have never been considered is that the trampoline has never been considered as an exercise device. Trampolines were considered as platforms for doing tricks.

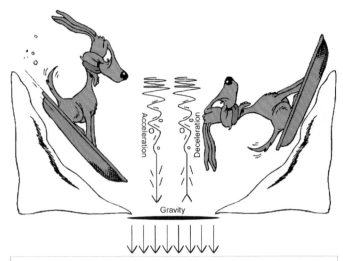

When rebounding the forces of acceleration and deceleration are lines up with the natural acceleration force of gravity. This stacks three different forces at the bottom of the bounce and causes an increase in the amount of gravity the body experiences.

When one performs on the trampoline he plays with gravity and the forces of acceleration and deceleration. To begin bouncing, a quick shove into the mat with both feet will force the trampoline bed downward until the tension of the bed and the extended springs is greater than the combined downward force of gravity and acceleration. The springs contract and the body is accelerated into the air. The next bounce includes the weight of the body along with the added force of acceleration as the body increases in velocity towards the center of the earth. The body lands on the mat and deceleration comes into play. Shoving the feet into the mat at the bottom of the bounce will force the trampoline to catapult the body to a greater altitude than before. Soon, enough altitude is gained so the trampolinist can begin somersaults and twists and other gymnastic moves.

From my experience trampolinists are not at all interested in any form of exercise. They just want to bounce. The reason they are not interested in exercise is because they simply don't need it. They are already strong well-balanced athletes. There was, however, a time and a place that the trampoline was used strictly for exercise. It happened at NASA.

NASA Experiments with Rebound
Exercise even before it Existed

"It's crazy, but it works," said C. E. (Pat) Mueller, thirty year director of Recreational Sports at the University of Minnesota.

"I've seen a lot of sports fads come and go," said Mueller, an associate professor with a master's degree in Physical Education. *"But this thing is so, phenomenal, it's the exercise of the future."*

One of the libraries I frequented as I did my research was the University of Washington. As I was going through the microfiche one day I found what Professor Mueller was referring to. The word "trampoline" was under the main heading, "NASA." Curious to find what NASA would be doing with a trampoline, I pulled the research and I am glad I did. NASA actually did research on the possibility of using a trampoline to help strengthen astronauts after space flight.

The Biomechanical Research Division, NASA-Ames Research Center, Moffett Field, California performed the research, in cooperation with the Wenner-Gren Research laboratory, University of Kentucky, Lexington, Kentucky.

The four scientists, A. Bhattacharya, E. P. McCutcheon, E. Shvartz and J. E. Greenleaf, secured the assistance of eight young men between the ages of 19 and 26 to each walk, jog and run on a treadmill which was operated at four different speeds and then jump on a standard sized trampoline at four different heights to compare the difference between the two modes of exercise.

Although treadmill running had been studied many times before, the scientists found that "...measurements of the necessary variables have not been reported previously for trampoline exercise." The trampoline testing was conducted at least one week after the treadmill testing.

The six measurements that were to be taken on all eight of the subjects while running on a treadmill and jumping on a trampoline were:

1. A pulse before exercising.
2. A pulse immediately after exercising.
3. The amount of oxygen consumed while exercising.
4. The amount of G-Force experienced at the ankle while exercising
5. The amount of G-Force experienced at the lower back while exercising.
6. The amount of G-Force experienced at the forehead while exercising.

The pulse would be obtained by a battery powered electrocardiograph unit taped to the subject's body which would transmit its signals to a custom designed receiver which in turn would record the information by electronically writing it on a chart. The oxygen consumption was to be measured with a K-meter that the subject would carry on his back. The G-Force experienced by the ankle, back and forehead of each of the university students would be measured by small sensitive accelerometers which would be placed in Plexiglas® holders and taped to the ankle, the small of the back and the forehead.

After thorough medical examinations, the healthy students were issued a pair of shorts and new Nike® running shoes to standardize their exercise conditions. They were then given familiarization sessions on laboratory procedures, treadmill running and trampoline jumping to ensure their exercise techniques would be the same. Each student then walked or ran four different speeds on the treadmill with a five to ten minute rest period between runs. Scientists recorded each student's statistics and compared the statistics with those of previous treadmill studies.

A week later, these same athletes returned to bounce on a trampoline at four different heights with a five to ten minute rest period in between exercise sessions. Again the scientists recorded each student's statistics. This time, they had no previous studies to compare them with. The results of trampoline vs. treadmill study were startling to the scientists.

I was ecstatic! Finally I had found a credible scientific study that confirmed what I was saying as a participating trampolinist. This wasn't just any study though, this was conducted by some of the world's best scientists. The following is information from NASA's findings. The indented statements are quotes from the study. The paragraphs are my explanations of the quotes."The G-Force measured at the ankle was always more than twice the G-Force measured at the back and forehead while running on a treadmill."

When a person runs, the back and head are usually fairly stationary. The legs and feet receive most of the musculoskeletal trauma of hitting a hard unforgiving surface. This information helps us better understand runners' injuries. Common injuries such as shin splints and knee problems are caused by intense trauma to the legs and feet while running. Injuries are especially prevalent when the natural shock absorbing system of the body becomes too fatigued to do its job correctly. This fatigue throws added strain on already tired muscles, bones, ligaments and tendons, often forcing them beyond the rupture point.

> "While jumping on a trampoline, the G-Force was almost the same at all three points, (ankle, back, forehead) and well below the rupture threshold of a normal healthy individual."

The surface of the trampoline is forgiving. The entire body, not just the lower extremities, shares the G-Force impact. This makes it possible to exercise the entire body without causing undue pressure to any part of the body. Also, each part of the body is receiving the necessary environmental stresses it needs to become stronger.

> "The external work output at equivalent levels of oxygen uptake was significantly greater while trampolining than running. The greatest difference was about 68%."

Rebounding efficiently uses the vertical forces of acceleration and deceleration to produce internal loading by directly opposing the gravitational pull. This develops more biomechanical work with less energy expended. Less oxygen is used and less demand is placed on the heart while stimulating the whole body.

> "While trampolining, as long as the G-Force remained below 4Gs, the ratio of oxygen consumption compared to biomechanical conditioning was sometimes more than twice as efficient as treadmill running...With the G-Force the same as or greater than 4Gs ...there was no significant difference in the oxygen uptake between the two regimens."

It is important to note that although this experiment was performed on a trampoline where the participants were able to develop a G-Force as high as 8Gs, the efficient use of energy was below 4Gs. People involved in rebounding on rebounders have been measured only as high as 3.5Gs, (see United States Air Force, Dr. Ward Dean, below) so that any activity on a rebound unit is more efficient than treadmill running at any speed.

"...averting the deconditioning that occurs during the immobilization of bed rest or space flight, due to a lack of gravireceptor stimulation (in addition to other factors), requires an acceleration profile that can be delivered at a relatively low metabolic cost...for equivalent metabolic cost and acceleration profile from jumping [on a trampoline] will provide greater stimuli to gravireceptors."

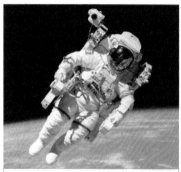

Rebounding is an effective method for rehabilitating astronauts who can lose large amounts of bone mass during space flight.

Rebound exercise is an excellent exercise for senior citizens, the physically disabled and those who are recuperating from space flight or injuries. It is also perfect for anyone else who needs exercise but is hampered by a preexisting condition.

"...for similar levels of heart rate and oxygen consumption, the magnitude of the biomechanical stimuli is greater with jumping on a trampoline than with running, a finding that might help identify acceleration parameters needed for the design of remedial procedures to avert deconditioning in persons exposed to weightlessness."

Now, if you are like me you had to read that scientific conclusion several times to even come close to what they were trying to say. But it is there. Rebounding is two to four times as efficient as treadmill jogging. Even people who are weak, bed ridden or exposed to weightlessness can and should rebound.

Chapter Six

Trampolining is Not the Answer, but Rebounding Just Might Be

From my biased point of view, in a perfect world everyone would have a full sized Olympic Style trampoline and everyone in the world would learn how to perform all of the basic trampoline gymnastic moves. Besides being fun it would be extremely beneficial to the health and strength of everyone.

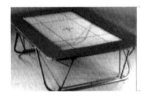

Trampolines can be fun to jump on and can be great for gymnastics. They are not ideal exercise for everyone however, because of the very high G-Force (up to 8 G's) the body can experience while jumping.

We don't live in my perfect world. Not everyone would want to do trampoline tricks even if they had the opportunity. A large trampoline needs space, either in a gymnasium or in the back yard. If it is in the back yard, it is subject to the inclement weather. Only a true trampolinist would want to jump on a trampoline while it is snowing. Besides, a person does not need to do tricks to receive the benefits of rebounding. What a person needs is a small round exercise device that is designed for rebound exercise. No tricks—just exercise. It should be small enough to fit in the front room or family room, and strong enough to handle the weight of all participants who are going to use it.

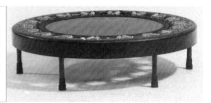

The Ultimate Rebound is a rebounder which folds into quarters. Its light weight composite polymer frame combined with its compact folding ability make it the most innovative rebounder on the market.

I first met Major Ward Dean, M.D., United States Air Force, over the telephone. He had just read my newly published book, *The Miracles of Rebound Exercise*, and decided he didn't like some of the things I had said. His major complaint was that I was making statements not supported by scientific studies and documentation.

"Sure, I can handle criticism," I remember saying. He then spent the next ninety minutes telling me what was wrong with my book, but to my surprise it was mostly punctuation and grammatical errors. Personally, I was devastated. That telephone conversation left me weak. To make things worse, I received a letter a week later enumerating, page by page, paragraph by paragraph, the many fallacies of my work. I did study his suggestions and corrected the mistakes in the book during subsequent printings.

I was surprised one day when Dr. Dean called me and asked me what he could test in his laboratory in Korea.

"Tell me how many Gs a person can develop on a rebounder. I need to know how safe it is."

"Okay." He said, "It's as good as done."

Near the end of January 1983, I received a copy of his Master's Thesis for his Master's Degree in Physiology from Kyungbook University, College of Medicine in Taegu, Korea. The subject?

"How much G-Force can be developed by an athlete in good physical condition bouncing on a quality rebounder at maximum attainable altitude."

His conclusion was approximately 3.24Gs. Trampolinists are able to handle 8Gs and do it many times during practice and competition, but the average person could be injured when exposed to such a large G-Force.

In chapter VIII of *Medical Physiology*, entitled, "Space Physiology," Guyton points out that the normal human can handle as much as 8Gs momentarily and 20Gs in a sitting position before vertebral fractures occur. "If the transverse acceleration forces are applied uniformly over large areas of the body, as much as 15–25 Gs can be withstood."

So, if the best athletes can develop only 3.24Gs, on a rebounder, rebounding is a safe whole body exercise for virtually everybody.

I guess the question of safety has to be an important one, especially since every book on exercise has one or two chapters on injury, everything from dog bites to shin splints.

This is probably what prompted Craig McQueen, M.D., to ask A. W. Daniels, Ph.D., Adjunct Professor, Material Science and Engineering and Orthopedic Surgery of the University of Utah, to analyze the comparison of the impact loads transmitted by rebounding and more conventional exercise surfaces.

In this report, they compared rebounding on a small rebounder to jogging on a hardwood basketball floor. Briefly, they accomplished the following:

They determined the approximate spring constant of the rebounder by measuring the deflection of the surface when various persons of known weight stood on it. It was found that the constant was 770 lb/ft.

They calculated the length of time of impulse load contact for a "typical" 165 lb. person running on a rebounder and on a hardwood basketball floor where the constant was 33,000 lb/ft. The time of contact with the mat or floor is inversely proportional to the impact force. The calculated times of contact were .13 seconds for the rebounder and .02 seconds on the floor.

Since .02 is only about 15% of .13, thus the maximum impact force on the rebounder would be only 1/6th that of the floor. The conclusion was that rebounding eliminates as much as 7/8[ths] or 87.5% of the trauma to the feet, knees and legs.

One of the major problems runners have is structural damage caused by the constant pounding of the skeleton against unforgiving surfaces. Peter Daetwiler of Hong Kong, an executive of a hotel chain, was a runner who needed weekly cortisone shots in his knee to combat pain and swelling. Then he was turned on to rebound exercise. He found he was able to main-

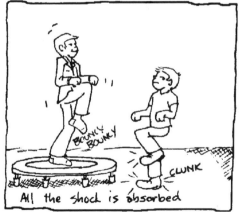

All the shock is absorbed

tain his level of cardiovascular endurance in the safety and convenience of his home in less time. He was also able to do it without the expensive and painful medication.

Since that time (1980) the springs on today's quality rebounders have been improved so dramatically that the latest quality rebounders may eliminate as much as 90% of the trauma to the lower extremities!

For a moment let us imagine rebound exercise has finally caught on and rebounding has become as well known as running or lifting weights. And everyone has access to rebounders. We all accept the fact, that the most efficient and effective way to harness the constantly available forces of acceleration and deceleration is to line them up with gravity. We readily accept that as the purpose of the rebounder. But children still do not understand why big people like to rebound for exercise. So, you explain to them,

"Children, please follow along closely. As you stand still on the rebounder, all parts of your body are subject to the force of gravity. This can be measured with a "G" meter. Are you familiar with a "G" meter?"

"Some say 'Yes,' others say 'No'."

You continue. "You probably have a "G" meter in your own home."

"I do?" Asks Billy.

"You may call it a bathroom scale."

"My mommy has one in our bathroom," Cindy volunteers.

"If you were to put a bathroom scale on top of a rebounder and stand on it, it would register the amount of G-Force the earth was pulling down on your entire body. One G-Force would be your total weight."

"I weigh 50 pounds," little Danny pipes up.

"I weigh 54," Hosea brags.

"However, something fascinating happens when you start jumping."

"Jumping is fun." interrupts Danny.

"At the bottom of the bounce, your whole body stops. You no longer weigh 1G you weigh more! That's deceleration. All body parts experience that G loading. Then, your body changes direction and increases in speed upward. That's acceleration."

As you bounce up and your feet leave the mat, your body begins to slow down because of the effect of gravity. You come to a complete momentary stop at the top of your free flight. At that moment you are weightless because the force of deceleration that is slowing your upward movement is directly opposite to and equal to the force of gravity. When you start down, you accelerate until your feet sink into the mat enough to cause the springs to slow you down. Your whole body feels the effects of acceleration and deceleration an average of two hundred times a minute! At the bottom of the bounce your body reacts to this environmental stimulation the same way it reacts to any other environmental change. All parts of your body adjust by becoming collectively stronger or more efficient in their specific function.

The reason NASA carried out the study of trampolining in the first place is because our astronauts lost as much as 14% of their muscle mass in fifteen days of space flight. The mice with a faster metabolism lost as much as 40% in the same period. They were suffering from deconditioning and osteoporosis, the same as the aged or the bedridden. NASA was looking for a non-traumatic form of exercise that would help to recondition a deconditioned astronaut. Can we assume the accepted forms of exercise were not acceptable to NASA? This is the only reason they would reach out from the accepted into new and unique forms of exercise never before considered.

Go to your local health club, athletic department or university. Listen to the athletic trainers as they explain to you how to use the various exercise equipment. As you read the messages on the side of the machines or work stations you will realize each machine is designed for exercising only a very specific set of the muscles of the body. Be aware, it is necessary to use many different machines to exercise all of the skeletal muscles. See if you can find an exercise machine designed to strengthen your skeleton. You will find none. Then look for the machine that is supposed to strengthen the involuntary muscles of your digestive system or your elimination system. I have not been able to find that machine.

Today's accepted exercise methods are not complete for an astronaut's body that just returned from a weightless environment, because they are not complete for any body. What NASA needs and was looking for is a whole body exercise—one that would strengthen the whole body all at once. And if it just happens to be more efficient, so be it.

Rebound Exercise is a Whole Body Exercise

The concept of a whole body exercise is new, with rebounding. It is refreshing and goes completely against the accepted forms of exercise presented to the general population by today's experts.

"There is no such thing as a utopic exercise that can be used to exercise the whole body! Or if there is, it certainly isn't suited for everybody." I have heard that for the last two decades. This statement usually comes from those who do not take the time to study the claims made by rebound exercise advocates. We have already established the common denominator of all exercises is opposing gravity. Let us establish another simple irrefutable fact.

44

All humans are made up of cells, about 100 trillion for each human body. That number is reached when a child reaches the age of two months. From that time on, every time a cell dies it is replaced by another cell. Although there are over two hundred different types of cells in the human body, all cells live in the same environment. That environment is water, nutrients, metabolic waste and gravity. Even the skin cells rely upon water received

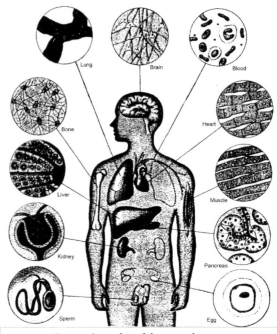

Here are just a few of the more than 200 different kinds of cells in the human body.

from within the body. If you want soft, supple, durable skin more able to resist germs and bacteria, be sure to drink plenty of water. The nutrients you take in through the mouth and the digestive system are distributed to all of the cells of the body. So far there is no argument, but when I include gravity as part of the cells' environment I begin to get a few eyebrows rising to the occasion.

Lift your hand up in front of you, then relax the muscles in you arm and watch it fall to your side as gravity pulls it down. If you are sitting while reading this book, chances are you are opposing gravity with the use of your arms, hands and finger muscles by holding the book up in front of you. You are also sitting upright because of the automatic behavior of the antigravity muscles of your abdomen and back that allow you to sit in your chair. If you were to go unconscious you would immediately fall out of your chair to the floor. Gravity will have its way unless you fight back.

Chapter Seven

The Philippines, My Medical Audience

Near the end of April 1983, I received an invitation from Mrs. Marcos, the First Lady of the Philippines, to go and do the same thing there that I had done in Hong Kong. So, my new flight arrangements back to the States included a one week visit to the "country of a thousand islands."

As I got off the airplane, I noticed a small contingent of military personnel waiting at the gate. What a surprise when I found out the military escort was waiting for me. As soon as I was identified one of the guards stepped forward and placed a nut lei around my neck. I was told to move to the center of the formation and with four military men in front and four behind me marching two abreast, we marched smartly right through customs to a waiting limousine. Although we didn't dally along the way, my luggage was already in the trunk by the time we arrived curbside.

I am easily impressed. They didn't have to do it, but it was an experience I'll never forget. With two motorcycles and a secret service automobile in front of the limo and the same behind, I was delivered to my luxury hotel in Manila. The flowers and fruit basket in my room were only a token of how I was to be pampered during my stay.

The next day, I was given a tour of the university built and donated by Mrs. Marcos to the youth of her country. This lovely hostess did everything she could possibly do to make my visit a memorable experience. Later that day, I was escorted to the palace where in the presence of her personal physician, my visit with Mrs. Marcos lasted an hour and a half. During this time I extolled the virtues of rebounding as clearly as I could.

"What's your opinion? " Mrs. Marcos asked her doctor.

"This is something I believe all medical doctors need to hear," was his surprising reply.

"That's just what I was thinking," she replied. "Will you make the arrangements?"

"Yes, Ma'am." He bowed, then turned to me. "Mr. Carter, would Thursday afternoon at one o'clock be all right with you?"

Completely flustered, I blurted, "I am at your service." What did I get myself into?

That was Tuesday. I spent all day Wednesday preparing for the meeting by going to their medical library and reserving their copy of *Medical Physiology* by Arthur C. Guyton, M. D., Morris's *Human Anatomy,* edited by J. Parsons Shaeffer and several other books in their library I hadn't seen before. If I had any chance at all to impress the doctors. I was going to have to meet them on their turf with their books so, I spent most of the night with my nose in the books searching for conclusive evidence that would keep me from being called a quack.

I was at the hospital before noon on Thursday checking out the lecture hall. It had a well lit stage two feet high and ten feet deep across the front of the room. I requested, and immediately got, a wireless lapel mike tuned into the state of the art in-house public address system. The room was set up for two hundred people. I was hoping for twenty-five.

At 12:45, the first of what was to be an audience of seventy-five nurses and fifty medical doctors began to arrive and take their seats. I selected three nurses and invited them to sit at a table next to the stage. I placed the books I had selected the day before in front of them and gave them instructions to look up and read what I asked them to read when I asked them to read.

The closer it got to 1:00, the more I began to realize the importance of this meeting. This was the acid test of the many theories of rebound exercise. If I were going to be shot down, this audience would be able to do it.

Was I ready to handle the humiliation if they got up and walked out?

What if I couldn't answer their questions to their satisfaction?

Do they believe in lynching foreign "quacks?"

Maybe I should walk out. I wondered how far it was to the airport. At 1:05, the doors closed.

Too late.

They made my introduction too flowery. Where did they get all that information about me anyway? Through the buzzing in my head I heard,

".... in for a unique experience. Please welcome, Dr. Albert Carter."

I'm no doctor, I thought, as I shifted mental gears from my personal pessimism to my public optimism. I reached to the back of my belt and turned on my wireless microphone as I moved center stage. I remember my presentation to that elite audience as if it happened yesterday.

"Thank you. I see you've done your homework, however, I'm not a doctor. I am a trampolinist and an author. I write about trampolining. I am here in front of you because something I said to Mrs. Marcos was valuable enough to her to cause her to request this meeting." Notice I blamed her just in case they didn't like what I said to them.

"Today, we are going to talk about the health benefits of exercise. I am not going to talk about your need for exercise, because I'm sure you already know how important exercise is to the overall health of the human body. In the next few minutes, I am going to introduce to you a form of exercise that, until recently, has been completely overlooked. It's an activity that has been around for over fifty years in the United States but has never been considered by our experts as an exercise. This activity is known as rebound exercise, the same type of exercise you would receive if you had access to a trampoline.

"A basic understanding of how all exercise affects the body will help you understand rebound exercise...."

I remember establishing the common denominator of all exercise is opposition to the gravitational pull of the earth. This caught their attention, because they had never thought of exercise in this light. Exercise has always been used to stimulate muscles. When I pointed out that the forces of acceleration and deceleration were facts of life but we had not taken advantage of them when it came to exercise, they became emotionally involved with the discussion.

"The vertical stacking of these three forces by rebounding has got to be one of the greatest breakthroughs in health maintenance!" I remember surprising even myself by making that statement. I backed it up by explaining that rebounding is a cellular exercise. We were no longer concerned about stimulating only the muscle fibers to greater strength, but every cell in the body. This included bone, nerve and connective tissue cells. There is no reason to believe this cellular stimulation does not include even the vital organs and hormone producing organs of the endocrine system.

I demonstrated the various forms of rebound exercise as I lectured. They applauded the aerobic exercises, and were amazed at the simplicity of the strength exercises. But I believe I made the greatest impact when I began to talk about the lymphatic system.

"You all know where the blood pump is. The heart starts beating before you are born and continues to beat until you die. But it only pumps blood. It does not pump lymph fluid. You have three times as much lymph fluid in your body as you do blood. Lymph fluid surrounds the tissue cells of the body. When the cells of the body need nutrients, they have to get it from the lymph fluid. When they excrete metabolic waste, it goes into the lymph. Obviously the more circulation your lymph fluid receives, the healthier you are going to be.

"The problem is we have never taken this mystifying system seriously. For example, we are able to hear the heart, measure the beat and monitor the pressure of the blood. But, because the lymphatic system just quietly goes about its job, not making waves, we don't study it.

"In fact, we have done just the opposite. Because we don't understand its importance, we have tried to get rid of it. We started forty years ago by removing the tonsils and the adenoids from healthy children, two of the drainage organs of the lymphatic system. We have no love for the appendix, another lymphatic drainage organ. Removal is in order every time a surgeon gets close to one. Lymph veins are stripped from the arms during a mastectomy. Until recently, the lymphatic system was just a big bother to the surgeon.

"A description of the lymphatic system will help you understand how rebounding actually multiplies the day to day function of this extremely important system."

I turned to the first of the three nurses sitting at the table and asked, "Would you please turn to page 361, in *Medical Physiology,* and read the very first paragraph of Chapter 31, the chapter on the lymphatic system?"

I spent the next half hour sweating profusely and explaining to medical doctors and nurses the importance of the lymphatic system and how rebound exercise stimulated this diffused organ of the human body.

Now came the scary part. I actually opened up the lecture for questions and answers. But, as a method of self-defense, every time a question was asked from the floor, I turned to my table of nurses and books and asked one of them to read the answer to the audience.

Question: "Mr. Carter, How do you know that exercise, and more specifically rebounding, has any effect on the immune system?"

Answer: "Thank you. To answer that, we need to know the relationship between the lymphatic system and the immune system." I turned to my nurse panel and asked, "Would you please turn to page 60 of *Medical Physiology* by Arthur C. Guyton and read the first two sentences?"

The first nurse took the book and spoke into the microphone. "The human body has the ability to resist almost all types of organisms or toxins that tend to damage the tissues and organs. This capacity is called immunity. Much of the immunity is caused by a special immune system that forms antibodies, and activated lymphocytes that attack and destroy the specific organisms and toxins. This type of immunity is acquired immunity. However, an additional portion of the immunity results from general processes. This is called innate immunity."

"Thank you. Now, continue with the third paragraph of the second column of the same page," I requested of my reader.

She continued, "We shall see that both the antibodies and the activated lymphocytes are formed in the lymphoid tissues of the body."

"To find out where the lymphoid tissue is found, read the first line of the fourth paragraph of page 61," I requested.

The soft voice continued, "The lymphoid tissue is located most extensively in the lymph nodes."

Question: "Mr. Carter, I thought the T-lymphocytes were manufactured in the Thymus and the B-lymphocytes were manufactured in the bursa, or bone marrow. Can you explain the apparent discrepancy?"

Answer: "Actually, both types of lymphocytes are derived originally in the embryo from pluripotent hemopoietic stem cells. After which, they receive further education or preprocessing from the thymus or bursa, but to answer where they go afterwards, turn to page 62, fourth paragraph."

Again the nurse read, "After formation of processed lymphocytes in both the thymus and the bursa, these first circulate freely in the blood for a few hours, but then become entrapped in the lymphoid tissue."

"So, you see, the activated lymphocytes and the antibodies whether manufactured by the T-lymphocytes or manufactured by the B-lymphocytes are sent out into the rest of the body from the lymph nodes. The speed with which they are dispatched is dependent on the speed of the lymph flow through the lymph nodes. If I could increase this function by 10–50 fold by exercising, I would make sure to do it daily."

Question: "Are you trying to tell us rebounding makes many medicines obsolete?"

Answer: "Not I. I am not a doctor so, I do not have the authority to say such things. Let's turn to the book all medical doctors have accepted as authoritive and see what it says. First, we need to understand the immune system's first and second lines of defense." Turning again to the nurses at the table, I asked, "Please read the second column on page 56 beginning with, 'The Tissue Macrophages'."

Again the microphone picked up the soft voice of a nurse. "The macrophages that are already present in the tissues immediately begin their phagocytic action. Therefore, they are the first line of defense against infection during the first hour or so. However, their numbers are not very great."

I continued, "I'm sure you will agree with me that the macrophages are the same cells as the monocytes. The only difference is the monocytes are immature cells freshly formed in the bone marrow and found in the bloodstream. As soon as they leave the bloodstream through the small holes in the capillary walls, they swell to five times their original size and become macrophages capable of destroying hundreds of bacteria by eating them. Now, read the following paragraph," I asked the same nurse. And she continued.

"Neutrophilia means an increase in the number of neutrophils (or white blood cells) in the blood. Within a few hours after the onset of acute inflammation, the number of neutrophils in the blood sometimes increases as much as four to five fold to as high as 15,000–25,000 per cubic millimeter."

"Thank you. Recall, if you will, that the neutrophils are only one fifth the size and capability of the macrophages, but usually out number them about ten to one.

"Now, please turn to page 57, and read the second paragraph."

The book was passed down to the third nurse. She read, "Almost any factor that causes some degree of tissue destruction will cause neutrophilia. For instance, persons debilitated by cancer exhibit an increase in neutrophils from the normal of 4500 per cubic millimeter sometimes up to 15,000 or more."

"That's good." I said. "Now read the fourth paragraph of the same column."

She continued, "The number of neutrophils in the circulatory system can increase as much as two to three times normal after a single minute of extremely hard exercise."

"Good. And the next paragraph." I was closing in for the kill and I could feel it.

"Approximately one hour after physiological neutrophilia has resulted from exercise, the number of neutrophils in the blood is usually back to normal."

"Do the neutrophils remain in the bloodstream?" I asked the audience.

"No." a doctor volunteered.

"Please explain." I requested.

"All lymphocytes have the ability to leave the blood stream by diapedesis, or squeezing through holes smaller than they are, and travel to the source of infection by chemotaxis."

Then I asked, "Once they leave the bloodstream, where are they?"

"In the extracellular fluid surrounding the cells." I heard from several of the nurses.

Question: "The concept of cellular exercise is intriguing because we have only thought of exercising groups of muscles. Do you have any reason to believe the individual lymphocytes actually become stronger, thereby making it faster and easier for the lymphocytes to get to the scene of the infection or injury?"

Answer: "That is a very good question. I have two references. First, let's see what gives the muscle the ability to contract. Please turn to Chapter Eleven, page 120, 'The Contraction of the Skeletal Muscle,' and read the first paragraph."

Again a soft honey voice was enhanced by the public address system. "Approximately 40% of the body is skeletal muscle and almost another 10% is smooth and cardiac muscle. Many of the same principles of contraction apply to all these different types of muscle."

"Thank you. To find out what principles of contraction they are talking about, let's go to page 121, third paragraph."

The same voice continued, "Each muscle fiber contains several hundred to several thousand myofibrils, which in turn has lying side by side, about 1500 myosin filaments and 3000 actin filaments, which are large polymerized protein molecules responsible for muscle contraction."

"Are we agreed, then, that the ability of the muscle to contract is dependent upon the interaction of the actin and myosin molecules?"

There was a general agreement from the audience.

"And we do agree that exercise does strengthen muscles?" Again, there was a general nodding.

"Then, if you will, please turn to page 24, first paragraph and let's find out how lymphocytes move."

Another voice filled the room. "It is believed amoeboid locomotion is caused in the following way: The outer portion of the cytoplasm is in a gel state and is called the ectoplasm, whereas the central portion of the cytoplasm is in a solid state and is called endoplasm. In the gel are numerous microfilaments composed of actin, and also present are many myosin molecules that interact with the actin to cause contraction the same as occurs in muscle."

Question: "Mr. Carter. Do you have the whole book memorized?"
There was a roll of laughter with that preposterous question.

Answer: "Just the important parts. I've had to defend my position on cellular exercise for so long that it became necessary to be prepared. Now, if cellular exercise is a valid concept, then scientists will come up with the same conclusion. Let me refer you to a study published in the *Physiologist Magazine*, December 1977."

Again, I turned to the table and asked, "What is the title of the study you have in front of you?"

"'Human Lymphocyte Activation is Depressed at Low G and Enhanced at High G.'"

"How many doctors involved with the study?" I asked my panel.

"Seven," came the immediate reply.

"Where did it take place?"

"Zurich."

"What lymphocytes were involved?"

"They were taken from the cosmonauts and astronauts."

"How active were lymphocytes after space flight or low G?"

"About 50% of the control group at 1G."

"After spinning them around in a centrifuge creating an 8G environment for three days, how active were they compared to the control?"

"At least twice as active."

"In fact, it says, 'Analysis of the ultra structure by electron microscopy shows that at high G cells are more swollen and richer in vacuoles than at 1G.'"

"So, you see, it is entirely possible that cellular exercise does exist, and rebounding is that cellular exercise. Rebound exercise creates that high G environment necessary to increase the strength and activity of the individual lymphocytes. This increases the efficiency of the entire immune system both collectively and individually cell by cell."

A Gratifying Conclusion

The meeting lasted a total of two and a half hours. At the end, those who wanted more information mobbed me. To call it a success seems too tame, yet I know of no other way to describe the results.

"That was the greatest demonstration of subject comprehension I have ever seen!" exclaimed the Head Surgeon as he came up to thank me for my demonstration.

"Thank you. Coming from you, that is the greatest compliment I have ever received," I returned, seriously.

Chapter Eight

Reboundology Physiology

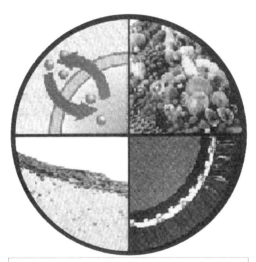

The four important aspects of maintaining a healthy cell are a favorable cell environment, nutritious cell food, clear cell communication and cell exercise.

Physiology is the study of functions in living matter. It attempts to explain the physical and chemical factors responsible for the development and progression of life. Each type of life from the very simple virus to the largest tree or even the human being has its own functional characteristics.

Therefore, the vast field of physiology can be divided into viral, bacterial, cellular, plant, animal and human physiology and many subdivisions.

In human physiology we attempt to explain the specific characteristics and mechanisms of the human body that make it a living being. The very fact we remain alive is almost beyond our own control. It is hunger that makes us seek food and fear that makes us seek refuge. Sensations of cold make us provide or search for warmth. Other forces cause us to seek fellowship and to reproduce. Thus the human being is actually an automation. The fact that we are sensing, knowledgeable beings is part of this automatic sequence of life. These special attributes allow us to exist under widely varying conditions that otherwise would make life impossible.

The Cell

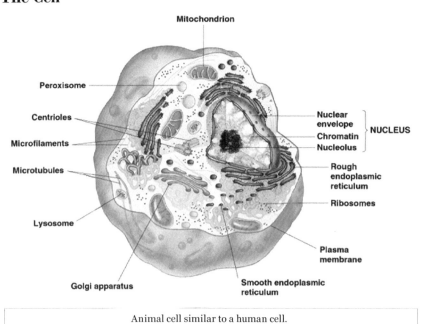

Animal cell similar to a human cell.

The basic unit of life in the body is the cell. Each organ, bone or system is an aggregate of many different cells held together by intercellular supporting structures. Each of the more than two hundred different types of cells is specially adapted to perform one particular function. For instance, one fourth of all the cells (approximately 25 trillion) are red blood cells. These cells are adapted to transport oxygen from the lungs to the tissues and carbon dioxide from the tissues back to the lungs.

Though the many cells of the body often differ markedly from each other, all of them have certain basic characteristics that are alike.

- In all cells, oxygen combines with carbohydrate, fat or protein to release the energy required for cell function.
- The general mechanisms for changing nutrients into energy are basically the same in all cells.
- All cells deliver the end products of their chemical reactions to the surrounding fluids.
- Almost all cells have the ability to reproduce. Whenever replenishable cells are destroyed, the remaining cells of that type divide again and again until the appropriate number is replenished.

So, cells are capable of living, growing and providing their special function so long as the proper concentrations of oxygen, glucose, amino acids, fats and the different ions are available to them in their environment.

A part of their environment that is overlooked is the ever present downward pull of gravity. It is overlooked because all humans, and therefore all human cells, experience approximately the same gravitational pull of the earth.

The cell is not merely a bag of fluid, enzymes and chemicals. It also contains highly organized physical structures called organelles. The physical nature of each of these is equally as important to the function of the cell as the cell's chemical constituents. For instance, without one of the organelles, the mitochondria, more than 95% of the energy supply of the cell would cease immediately.

The Cell is a Busy City

The activity inside one cell is hard to comprehend. In fact, as one doctor explained to me as we were sharing a flight coming into Chicago O'Hara Airport at five thousand feet, "Look as far as you can see in all directions. Imagine you are aware of every type of movement in Chicago regardless of where it is. As soon as you can comprehend all that activity, you will have an idea of the amount of activity going on inside each cell of your body at this very moment."

Our cells play an important part in nature. There are tens of billions of known organic molecules. Yet only about fifty of them are used by the cells of plants and animals in the essential activities of life. The same patterns are employed over and over again, conservatively, ingeniously for different functions of different cells.

In the living cell, fragments of food are miraculously changed into intricate cellular machinery. Inside it is a labyrinthine architecture that maintains its own structural strength, transforms molecules, stores energy and prepares for self-replication.

Volumes of books have been written about the human cells, but we are only going to talk about a few of the many parts.

If we could enter the fluid of a cell, the cytoplasm, we would find it is composed mainly of six basic substances: water, minerals, electrolytes, proteins, lipids and carbohydrates. Many of the molecular specks we would see would be protein molecules, some in frenzied activity, others merely waiting.

DNA, The Boss Molecules

Another thing that is usually overlooked is the amazing intelligence of each of the 100 trillion cells of the body. Almost everyone knows the genes control heredity from parents to children, but most people do not realize the same genes control the production of the day by day function of all cells. The genes control cell function by determining what substances will be synthesized within the cell—what structures, what enzymes, what chemicals and how strong the cell membrane has to be. These genes, or nuclear proteins found at the center of the cell, control cell chemistry and the nucleic acids that carry the hereditary instructions. We find these nuclear molecules (DNA or deoxyribonucleic acid) to be essentially identical in all plants and animals.

Understanding the DNA inside our cells is relatively new and is an ongoing process. DNA was first presented to the scientific world the same year John F. Kennedy was assassinated and finally mapped the same year the Twin Towers were destroyed. These nucleic acids are the boss molecules. They live sequestered behind the nuclear membrane deep in the nucleus of the cell city.

If we plunged through a pore into the nucleus of the cell, we would find something that resembles an explosion in a spaghetti factory, a disorderly multitude of coils and strands. These strands are comprised of tightly coiled DNA. DNA is a double helix. It's two intertwined strands resemble a "spiral" staircase. It has a sequence of nucleotides along either of the constituent strands. Nucleotides are the molecular components that make up DNA. The language of life is written in four letter code of these components. Information stored in the DNA of a whale or a vegetable is written in this same four-letter language.

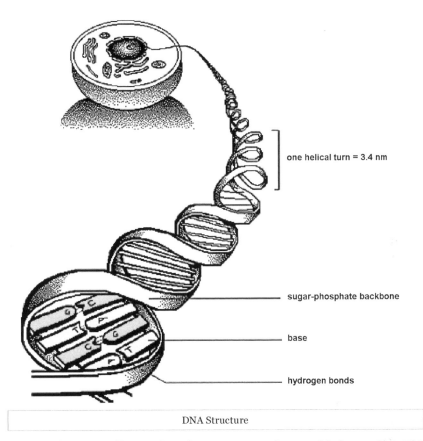

one helical turn = 3.4 nm

sugar-phosphate backbone

base

hydrogen bonds

DNA Structure

The human cell contains about 714 megabytes of information. This information is all stored on the DNA in the nucleus of each of our cells. If these DNA molecules were uncurled into a long straight line it would extend three feet. Every millimeter of the DNA strand is filled with the information that makes you you. In fact if all the information recorded in one DNA molecule was translated into English there would be enough information to fill four thousand volumes of books as thick as the Bible.

Still, our scientists do not understand the function of most of the DNA. Though there are very few nucleic acid molecules which are useful to humans, the number of useful ways of putting these nucleic acids together is stupefying. Some say the possible combinations are probably far greater than the total number of electrons and protons in the universe.

This is all of the information needed to make a cell or a human work. What is more, the DNA molecules know how to clone identical copies of

60

themselves with very few mistakes. In addition to making accurate copies of itself, DNA directs the activities of the cell. DNA is what directs metabolism by synthesizing another nucleic acid called messenger

RNA, The Messenger

There are two kinds of nucleic acids: DNA—deoxyribonucleic acid and RNA—ribonucleic acid. DNA knows what to do, and RNA conveys the instructions issued by DNA to the rest of the cell. DNA is found only inside the nucleus, and the construction of the protein molecules is performed outside the nucleus

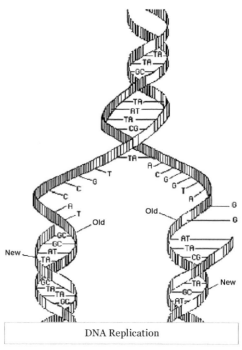

DNA Replication

by the ribosome. Because of this, the instructions on protein manufacture have to be delivered from the DNA to the ribosome. Transmitting these messages is the job of the RNA. It constantly travels from the DNA to the ribosome telling it what proteins to produce.

To provide the protein message accurately, the DNA unwinds to show the construction message to the RNA. Once the unwinding is underway, a remarkable enzyme called DNA polymerase helps ensure that the copying works almost perfectly. The RNA pairs up with one side of the DNA and reads the message of the protein to be produced. The RNA then releases itself from the DNA and floats out of the nucleus with the captured message.

Each messenger RNA passes to the extra-nuclear provinces, the cytoplasm. There they control the construction of protein.

The sequence of the RNA code is the identity of the protein that will be produced. At the ribosome the protein is assembled one nucleotide at a time (about ten per second). These nucleotide building blocks are found floating nearby in the cell's cytoplasm. If a mistake is made, there are enzymes, which snip the mistake out and replace the wrong nucleotide with the right one. When all is done a single protein molecule has been produced.

1. Transcription

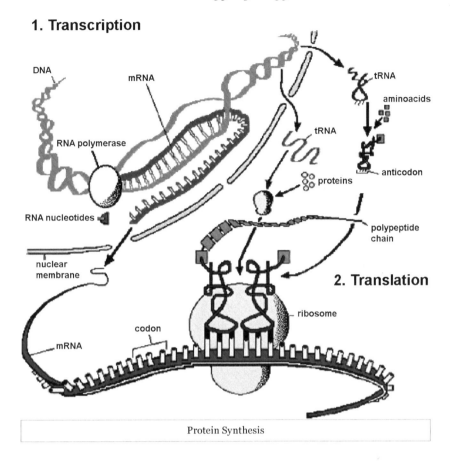

Protein Synthesis

Enzymes are Factory Workers

All of the proteins your body will ever need are manufactured inside the cells of your body under the direct information received by the RNA from the DNA. The most important proteins are enzymes (factory workers), molecules that control the cell's chemical reactions. These enzymes promote synthesis of lipids, glycogen, purines, pyrimidines and hundreds of other substances. Our cells know how to manufacture over 50,000 different enzymes for the millions of chemical reactions happening inside the cells daily. Enzymes are like assembly line workers, each specializing in a particular molecular job: such as the construction of one of four nucleotides, guanosine phosphate or the dismantling of a molecule of sugar to extract energy. But the enzymes are only factory workers. They do not run the show. They receive their instructions on orders sent from the DNA.

Every one of your one hundred trillion cells contains a complete library of instructions on how to make every part of them and you. Every cell in your body is created by successive cell divisions beginning with a single fertilized egg cell created by your parents. Every time that cell divided, in the many embryological steps that went into making you, the original set of genetic instructions was duplicated with great fidelity. So, your liver cells have some unemployed knowledge about how to make your bone cells, and vice versa. Your heart muscle cells know how to function as brain cells. The genetic library contains everything your body knows how to do on its own. This ancient information is written in exhaustive, careful, redundant detail. Instructions on how to laugh, sneeze, cry, walk, recognize patterns, reproduce, digest and how to adjust to different environments is all carefully recorded in the DNA of each of your 100 trillion little cells.

Technology can duplicate only a tiny fraction of the intricate biochemical reactions our bodies effortlessly perform. We have only just begun to study these processes, but one thing that is usually overlooked is that the very same DNA which controls our genetic make-up also controls our make-up on a cellular level.

Cellular Exercise?

Exercise experts readily acknowledge that muscle cells have the ability to automatically adjust to stressful exercise programs. What is not usually recognized is all other cells have the same capability. Stimulated bone cells become mineralized, dense and strong. An athlete's skin is thicker and more supple. Even the lymphocytes, the white blood cells of the immune system, are individually stronger when physically challenged. All cells of the body have the ability of automatically adjusting to their environment in their own specific way. Some cells adjust so dramatically that it is readily measurable. Others adjust so minutely that it is hard if not impossible to measure the change.

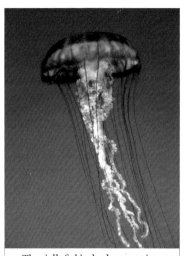

The jellyfish's body experiences less gravity while developing. When a jellyfish leaves the water and experiences gravity, it is completely unable to move because of the weakness of the cells.

The cell membrane of each and every cell has to be strong enough to keep from rupturing under normal environmental conditions such as one G-Force. It also must be flexible enough to allow movement and permeable enough to allow body fluid to move through the membrane in both directions.

The body of a jellyfish is made up of cells having the same basic functions as the cells in our bodies. The difference is that the jellyfish floats all its life in water. The buoyancy nullifies the force of gravity. When the jellyfish is taken out of the water it is unable to move. The cell membranes of the jellyfish rupture and die.

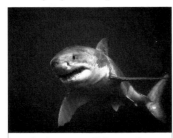

Sharks are terrifying predators, but because of their underwater lifestyle, their bodies fall apart with the pressures of gravity.

The shark is a mean predator. Its muscles are strong because they have to propel the shark through the water. The shark, like the jellyfish, does not have to oppose the force of gravity. This is why when the shark is caught by fishermen and hung up by its tail, the connective tissues that hold its organs inside are not strong enough and the organs fall out through its mouth, a self-cleaning shark.

All human cells have an outside surface called a cell membrane which is made up of 85% protein and 15% lipids. The thickness of each cell membrane is dependent upon how much stress is placed upon it. When extra stress is placed on a cell, DNA sends messenger RNA to the ribosomes to produce specific enzymes. Then these enzymes, responsible for keeping the cell membrane strong, immediately begin their complicated task.

The opposite of stress is no stress and the opposite of strength is weakness. The absence of gravity during the prolonged space flight of astronauts is a health concern for NASA. At 77, John Glenn, the first American to orbit the Earth nearly 40 years ago, went up into space once again. This time it was to help the National Institute on Aging (NIA).

"My interest in understanding what it is that happens to the body in zero gravity and what benefits that will have for the problems of aging," says Richard Sprott, associate director of the biology of aging at NIA, Bethesda, MD."The key point is that there is some genuine scientific interest between [NIA and NASA]."

Microgravity

Once in orbit, the space vehicle and everything inside it experiences a condition called microgravity. The vehicle and its contents appear to be weightless, floating inside the spacecraft. For this reason, microgravity is

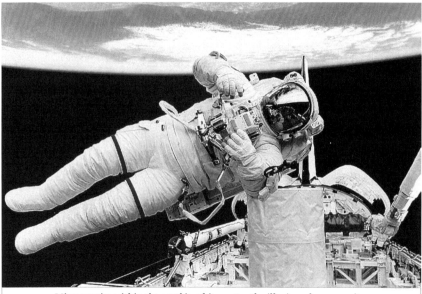

Microgravity within the earth's orbit creates the illusion of zero gravity.

also referred to as zero gravity. However, both terms are technically incorrect. The gravitation in orbit is only slightly less than the gravitation on the earth. The spacecraft and its contents continuously fall toward the earth, but because of the vehicle's tremendous forward speed, the earth's surface curves away as the vehicle falls toward it.

Microgravity has major effects on both equipment and people. For example, fuel does not drain from tanks in microgravity, so it must be squeezed out by high pressure gas. Hot air does not rise in microgravity, so fans must drive air circulation. Particles of dust and droplets of water float throughout the cabin only to settle in filters on the fans.

The human body reacts to microgravity in a number of ways. In the first several days of a mission, about half of all space travelers suffer from persistent nausea, sometimes accompanied by vomiting. Vomiting can be messy because the vomit does not fall to the floor, it sprays outward and only stops when it hits something. Most experts believe this "space sickness," called space adaptation syndrome, is the body's natural reaction to microgravity. Drugs to prevent motion sickness can provide some relief for the symptoms and the condition generally passes in a few days.

Microgravity also confuses an astronaut's vestibular system—that is, the organs of balance in the inner ear—by preventing it from sensing differences in direction. After a few days in space, the vestibular system disregards all directional signals. Soon after an astronaut returns to the earth, the organs of balance resume normal operation.

Over a period of days or weeks in space, an astronaut's body experiences deconditioning. In this process, the heart and blood vessels "get lazy," thus creating a decrease in maximum cardiac output because there is a decrease in blood volume.

In space, muscle cells go through the demineralization process causing a decrease in muscle strength and work capacity. Also, bones in space loose minerals causing osteoporosis. There is a decrease in the physical strength of the lymphocytes, reducing the efficiency of the immune system. Other effects of weightlessness, like thinning of the skin and weakening of the involuntary digestive muscles, are very probable but were not measured.

Because the muscle cells, connective tissue cells and bone cells become weaker, in fourteen days of space flight astronauts have been known to loose as much as 15% of bone and muscle mass. Space mice with a faster metabolism have lost up to 40% in the same period of time.

Muscles, connective tissues, bones, lymphocytes and skin become weaker because the cells of the entire body determine that physical strength is not necessary in a weightless environment. With less hydraulic pressure in the body it is easier to deliver oxygen to the cells. Less blood cells are produced because fewer are required. Essentially these same effects occur in people confined to bed rest.

It appears the cells of the body have a greater ability to adjust to their environment than what we give them credit for. Without gravity during space flight, the cells of the muscles take it upon themselves to adjust to their new environment. Did NASA find their space age exercise? It appears so. Rebounding appears to be a way of "averting the deconditioning that occurs during the immobilization of bed rest or space flight, due to a lack of gravireceptor stimulation (in addition to other factors)."

Their studies pointed out, "While trampolining, as long as the G-Force remained below 4Gs, the ratio of oxygen consumption compared to biomechanical conditioning was sometimes more than twice as efficient as treadmill running." Translation: rebounding uses less oxygen to produce more biomechanical conditioning when compared to running on the old fashioned treadmill.

Although this experiment was performed on a trampoline where the participants were able to develop a G-Force as high as 8Gs, it is important to note the efficient use of energy was below 4Gs. A study of rebound exercise accomplished by Dr. Ward Dean, M.D. of the United States Air Force proved rebounding is safe for most people.

So, is it possible for one to exercise all of the cells of the body all at once? The answer to that question is "yes." This is accomplished simply by jumping up away from gravity. At the moment one jumps vertically, all of the cells of the body experience both the forces of acceleration and gravity. Since the cells of the body have no idea what is happening, they just feel the sudden increase in the G-Force. To survive, all DNA molecules of all cells react sending messages through the RNA to produce more protein. This protein is added to the cell membrane to bolster its strength.

Once the inertia of the jump is expended, gravity takes over and pulls the body back to the Earth. Upon contact with the surface of the Earth the body experiences the combined forces of deceleration and gravity. More molecular messages are sent, and more adjustments at the cell level are made. Without a rebounder this jumping action does create a problem. When one lands on the hard surface of the unforgiving Earth the combined forces of gravity and deceleration could create a 15–20 G-Force at the feet, ankles, knees and hips. That might be beyond the rupture threshold of certain cells of the ankles, shins and knees, especially if this activity is done over and over again. It is possible that some of the cells in these areas will rupture and die. The body will experience bruising, internal hemorrhaging and shin splints—injuries experienced by even experienced runners and joggers.

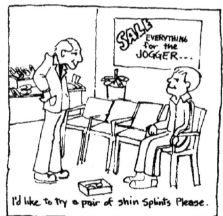

As presented by Dr. Ward Dean, jumping on a quality rebounder will reduce the extreme G-Force down to under 3Gs. This is well under the rupture threshold of all cells of the body. Because of this a person can immediately rebound again without the fear of injury. The participant's body benefits a hundred times a minute from the effects of a safely increased G-Force.

Combining the natural forces of acceleration and gravity vertically by rebounding challenges all cells. Most cells adjust to an increased G-Force and become stronger individually and the entire body becomes stronger collectively. Other cells which don't need to or aren't able to become stronger, simply become more efficient instead.

Suddenly we now have a whole body exercise that seems so simple. You see exercise methods like calisthenics, weight lifting or jogging, each individually exercise only specific parts of the body at a time. We are bombarded with television infomercials which extol the virtues of Gut Busters, Ab Flexors, Thigh Masters, Aerobic Rockers and the Health Rider. I am sure you have noticed testimonials are easy to come by. And rightly so, because if those exercise devices based on old-fashioned concepts are used, most people will receive strengthening benefits to that particular part of the body for which the exercise was designed.

Still, even the manufacturers of those exercise devices will tell you in order to exercise the entire body, you will have to use other pieces of equipment. May I suggest the use of a rebounder as the "other piece of equipment?" Rebounding is a cellular exercise because it causes all of the cells of the body to physically adjust to what is perceived by them as a more demanding internal environment.

We didn't ask their permission.

We just did it.

They have to adjust.

They have no choice.

Chapter Nine

Reliable Cellular Reactions
to Rebound Exercise

The Mitochondria— The Powerhouse of the Cell

Each of the more than two hundred different types of cells have unique jobs, but there are some jobs that all cells do the same. All cells import various products through the cell membrane. All cells export metabolic waste through the cell membrane. All cells produce various enzymes and hormones. They all carry on chemical reactions to accomplish their required tasks. Cells all need to import nutrients, export waste products and manufacture hormones. They must contract or expand depending on requirements, and carry on other cellular activities. Nerve cells send messages. Muscle cells move either various parts of the body or foodstuffs. Bone

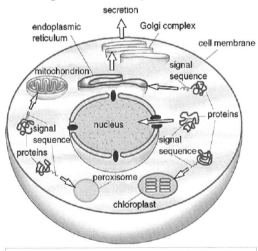

Each cell is bustling with hundreds of different activities, which help to maintain homeostasis in the body.

cells import and export bone mineral and deposit it around the outside of the cell membrane. All of these jobs require energy. All animal cells rely upon mitochondria to produce that energy.

Mitochondria (mitochondrion, singular) are the sources of 95% of all the energy required by the cells. That is why the mitochondria are called the "powerhouses of the cell." Without them the cells would be unable to extract significant amounts of energy from nutrients and oxygen, causing nearly all cellular functions to cease. These organelles are present in most areas of the cell's cytoplasm, but the number per cell varies from less than a hundred to several thousand, depending upon the amount of

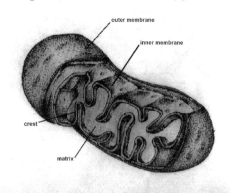

Mitochondria are the powerhouses of the cells. They produce energy that is used in all of the processes that the cells of the body perform.

energy required by each cell. Mitochondria are concentrated in those portions of the cell that metabolize the most energy. Mitochondria vary in size and shape; some are only a few hundred millimicrons in diameter and globular in shape while others are as large as one micron in diameter, as long as seven microns and filament like in shape. The basic structure of a mitochondrion is composed mainly of two lipid bilayer protein membranes: an outer membrane and an inner membrane.

The principal substances from which cells extract energy are oxygen and one or more of the foodstuffs—carbohydrates, fats and proteins. In the human body essentially all carbohydrates are converted into glucose or blood sugar *before* they reach the cell. The proteins are converted into amino acids, and the fats are converted into fatty acids. Inside the cell, the foodstuffs react chemically with oxygen. This reaction is facilitated by various enzymes which control the rate of reaction and channel energy that is released in the proper direction.

The many folds of the inner membrane form shelves or crests onto which oxidative enzymes are attached. Also, the inner cavity of the mitochondrion is filled with a gel matrix containing large quantities of the enzymes necessary for extracting energy from nutrients. These enzymes operate in association with the oxidative enzymes on the shelves. Together they oxidate nutrients forming carbon dioxide and water as by-products.

The liberated energy is made into a high energy substance called adenosine triphosphate (ATP). ATP is then transported out of the mitochondrion. This energy is then diffused throughout the cell and used wherever it is needed.

ATP (adenosine triphosphate)

ATP is a nucleotide composed of the nitrogenous base adenine, the pentose sugar ribose and three phosphate radicals. Two of the phosphate radicals are connected to the molecule with high-energy phosphate bonds. Each of these bonds contains about 12,000 calories of energy per mole of ATP under the physical conditions of the body (7,300 calories under standard conditions). This is much more energy than is stored in the average chemical bond of other organic compounds. That is why they are called "high-energy" bonds.

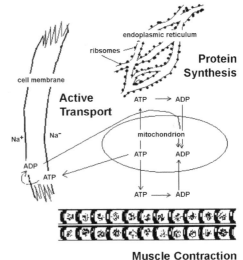

ATP is the vital energy currency which fuels muscle contractions and muscle synthesis.

Furthermore, the high-energy phosphate bond is very labile or unstable. It can be split instantly whenever energy is required. When ATP releases its energy, a phosphoric acid radical is split away, and adenosine diphosphate (ADP) is formed. Then, energy derived from the cellular nutrients causes the ADP and phosphoric acid to recombine to form new ATP, the entire process continues over and over again. ATP has been called the energy currency of the cell, because it can be spent and remade again and again.

The major portion of the ATP formed in the cell is formed in the mitochondria. The pyruvic and fatty acids and most of the amino acids are all converted into the compound acetyl-CoA in the matrix of the mitochondrion. This substance, in turn, is acted upon by a series of enzymes and undergoes dissolution in a sequence of chemical reactions called the citric acid cycle or Krebs cycle.

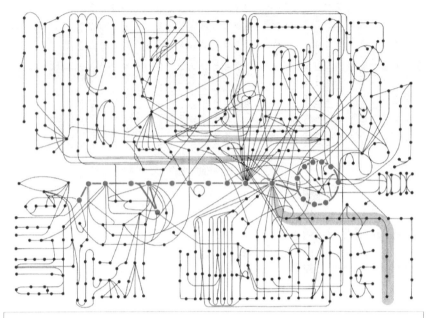

The Citric Acid Cycle (or Krebs Cycle) is a maze of chemical
reactions that convert ATP into energy.

Uses of ATP for Cellular Function

ATP energy currency is used to promote three major categories of cellular functions:

1) membrane transport,
2) synthesis of chemical compounds throughout the cell, and
3) mechanical work.

ATP is required for membrane transport of potassium ions and sodium. In certain cells calcium, phosphate, chloride, urate, hydrogen ions and many other substances are transported. Membrane transport is so important to cellular function that some cells, the renal tubular cells (in the kidneys) for instance, use as much as 80 per cent of the ATP they form for this purpose alone.

In addition to synthesizing proteins, cells also synthesize phospholipids, cholesterol, purines, pyrimidines and a great host of other substances. Synthesis of almost any chemical compound requires energy. For instance, a single protein molecule might be composed of as many as several thousand amino acids attached to each other by peptide bonds. The formation of each of these linkages requires the breakdown of three high energy bonds. Thus many thousand ATP molecules must release their energy as each protein molecule is formed. In fact, some cells utilize as much as 75% of all the ATP formed in the cell simply to synthesize new chemical compounds. This is particularly true during the growth phase of cells.

The final major use of ATP is to supply energy for special cells to perform mechanical work. Each contraction of a muscle fiber requires expenditure of tremendous quantities of ATP. Other cells perform mechanical work in two additional ways, by ciliary or amoeboid motion. The source of energy for all these types of work is ATP.

In summary, ATP is available to release its energy rapidly and almost explosively wherever and whenever the cell needs it. To replace the ATP used by the cell, other much slower chemical reactions break down carbohydrates, fats and proteins and use the energy derived from these to form new ATP. About 95% of this ATP is formed in the mitochondria, often called the "powerhouses" of the cell.

Human Endurance is a Function of the Cells

Why are we spending so much time on the mitochondria? Because it is a very unique part of the cell. It reacts to exercise, more specifically, rebound exercise. Mitochondria are the energy source that lights us up, cell by cell. They also have the unique ability to replicate themselves without permission from the DNA. Thus one mitochondrion can form a second one, a third one and so on, whenever there is need in the cell for increased amounts of ATP. The mitochondria contain a special type of deoxyribonucleic acid, its own DNA, similar to that found in the nucleus. This substance allows the mitochondrion to clone itself without receiving instructions from the nucleus. This replication is done whenever there is a need for increased production of cellular energy.

Why is this so important? Simply because human endurance is directly related to the number of these powerhouses in each cell. Because mitochondria are duplicated as needed, available energy is first used up before new mitochondria are created. This energy deficit sends a message to the mitochondria that more energy is required. The mitochondria then begin to replicate and next time the energy is required, a greater amount of energy will be available. The more mitochondria you have in the muscles you are using, the greater the endurance of those muscles.

Any exercise that depletes the ATP will help you to increase your endurance. But rebounding does the job more efficiently because ALL of the cells are being challenged at the very same time up to a hundred times a minute. That means ALL mitochondria are receiving the same message. *"Produce more energy—and if you can't do it by yourself, get help!"*

That is why a person who starts rebounding may be able to jump for only 30 seconds to a minute, but a week later find they are able to rebound more than ten minutes without getting tired. Soon they are rebounding for thirty minutes to an hour. By rebounding they have created energy to burn. This excess energy is now available to them all day long in virtually any human activity.

Space flight and bed rest reduce the number of mitochondria per cell. Less energy is required so, the cell dismantles the extra mitochondria. Rebounding causes all of the cells to expend energy and demand more energy all at once, dramatically increasing the number of mitochondria per cell. The increased number of mitochondria increase available energy to the cells and the whole body. This increases the endurance of the whole body.

Chapter Ten

The Musculoskeletal System

Muscle Contraction is a Function of the Cell

The next time you go to an exercise gymnasium, take a look at the side of the exercise equipment you use. It will show you what muscles that device or station is designed to challenge. Notice also that it doesn't say a thing about the muscle cells or how they contract. Is the ability to contract the property of the muscle or is it the property of the muscle cell?

About 40% of the body is skeletal muscle, and perhaps another 10 per cent is smooth and cardiac muscle. Many of the same principles of contraction apply to all these different types of muscle. So, we will present the function of the skeletal muscle. In most muscles, the muscle cells extend the entire length of the muscle. For example, the muscle cells in a giraffe's neck are seven feet long!

Each muscle cell is filled with many cell fibers that extend the length of the muscle cell. Each muscle fiber has a nerve cell connected near the middle of the fiber. Each muscle fiber contains several hundred to several thousand myofibrils. Each myofibril in turn has, lying side by side, about 1500 myosin filaments and 3000 actin filaments. These large protein molecules are responsible for muscle contraction.

The myofibrils are suspended inside the muscle fiber in a matrix called sarcoplasm. Sarcoplasm is composed of the usual intracellular constituents—potassium, magnesium, phosphate and protein enzymes. There is also a tremendous number of mitochondria filled with ATP to be used for muscle contraction.

How does a Muscle Contract?

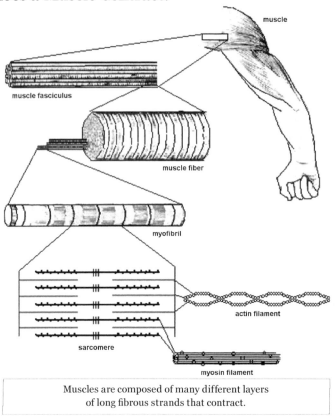

Muscles are composed of many different layers
of long fibrous strands that contract.

1. A neural message travels along a motor nerve to the middle of the muscle fiber.
2. The neural message secretes a small amount of acetylcholine.
3. The acetylcholine acts on the local area of the muscle fiber membrane to open multiple acetycholine-gated channels through protein molecules in the muscle fiber membrane.
4. Opening of the acetylcholine channels allows large quantities of sodium ions to flow to the interior of the muscle fiber membrane at the point of the nerve terminal. This stimulates the muscle fiber.
5. The neural message travels along the muscle fiber membrane in the same way that neural messages travel along nerve membranes.

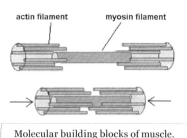

Molecular building blocks of muscle.

6. The neural message depolarizes the muscle fiber membrane and also travels deeply within the muscle fiber. There it causes the sarcoplasmic reticulum to release into the myofibrils large quantities of calcium ions that have been stored within the reticulum.

7. The calcium ions initiate attractive forces between the actin and myosin filaments, causing them to slide together, which is the contractile process.

8. After a fraction of a second, the calcium ions are pumped back into the sarcoplasmic reticulum, where they remain stored until a new muscle action potential comes along; this removal of the calcium ions from the myofibrils causes muscle contraction to cease.

Sound complicated? Chemically, it is, but it all happens in the blink of an eye, literally. Each time you blink an eye this entire process of contraction and relaxation occurs at the cell level. It also happens at exactly the right moment. The muscular movements of the fingers of a piano player or the muscular coordination of a basketball player, a long distance runner, a wrestler, a gymnast or a ballet dancer have to be precise and dependable every time. The necessary chemicals have to be pumped in and out of the muscle fibers hundreds of times a minute in order for an athlete to play his sport.

Rebound exercise enhances and challenges the delivery system of the chemicals of the muscle fibers every time one lands on the rebound mat surface.

Developing Muscle Mass is a Function of the Cells

The enlargement of muscle mass is called hypertrophy. The myofibrils themselves split within each muscle fiber to form new myofibrils. As a result of hypertrophy, all of the muscle chemicals required for muscle activity increase. This includes enzyme systems for fast energy conversion, calcium and ATP.

When the muscle mass becomes smaller this is atrophy. When a muscle remains unused for a long period of time the contractile protein decays more rapidly than it is replaced.

All the muscles of the body are continually being remodeled to match the functions required of them. Their diameters, lengths, strengths, vascular supplies and even the types of muscle fibers are altered. This remodeling process is often quite rapid, within a few weeks. Indeed, experiments have shown even under normal conditions, the muscle contractile proteins can be totally replaced in as little as two weeks.

The muscle contractile proteins we are talking about are the actin and the myosin filaments. It is relatively easy to achieve larger muscles, it just takes a few strong contractions. If you do as little as three sets of six contractions at close to maximal strength, every other day for six to ten weeks your muscles will hypertrophy.

Most people have no problem at all accepting the idea that rebounding develops large leg muscles, because they can see the physical activity in the legs. When I tell them rebounding builds larger arm muscles at the same time, they scratch their heads and ask, "Are you sure?"

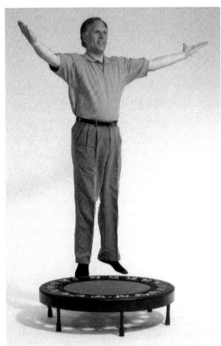

The biceps are perpendicular to the pull of gravity. This causes the biceps to oppose the increased G-Force at the bottom of the bounce by holding up the weight of the arm times the force of gravity experienced.

My answer, of course is, "Yes. I am sure, and I can prove it in less than a minute."

Here is my proof. Stand on a rebounder and extend one of your arms out horizontally in front of you with the palm of your hand up. With the other hand, put your thumb on the inside of the biceps and your fingers on the outside of the biceps of the extended arm. Now begin to bounce and notice that the biceps expand every time you land on the rebounder. The expansion you feel each time you land means the muscle is working. If you rebound with your arms extended horizontally until you can no longer hold them out, this will cause some of the myofibrils of the biceps to split and become two. Your biceps will become larger and stronger. You will be able to feel the difference in thickness of the biceps in as little as three days. A difference in strength will be noticeable in the same length of time.

The mitochondria are also being challenged, so the biceps will have more endurance. Now, isn't that exciting?

Now that we know this, let's use it. Stand on the rebounder with both arms out in front of you or to the side with the palms of your hands up and bounce. Do this for several minutes or until you feel the burn. You can exercise the triceps by extending your arms out horizontally in front or to the side with your thumbs pointing down. Bounce for several minutes until you feel the fatigue in your triceps. Add these simple routines to your rebounding. You might as well since you are going to be rebounding anyway.

It has long been taught that in order to achieve hypertrophy one must put the muscle in question through a full range of motion under stress many times. It is easy for a person to accept that supposition, because weight lifting does produce larger muscles. But what is surprising is consistent rebounding also increases muscle thickness of the upper body without necessarily putting the muscles through a full range of motion. The rebound action is created mostly by the calf muscles in the legs, however all of

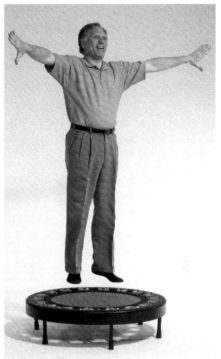

In this move the triceps are perpendicular to gravity. When the triceps oppose the increased G-Force, holding up the weight of the arm, the force of gravity increases that perceived weight.

the skeletal, smooth and even the cardiac muscles of the entire body accept rebounding as a challenge. They all begin to become stronger, thicker and more able to endure.

All Involuntary Muscles of the Digestive System are Strengthened by Rebounding

Skeletal muscles are used to move the body around in its environment by working with the bones of the skeleton. Skeletal muscles cells are as much as twenty times as large in diameter and thousands of times as long as the cells of the smooth muscles. Most importantly, many of the principles of contraction apply to smooth muscle cells the same way they apply to skeletal muscle cells. Essentially the same attractive forces between myosin and actin filaments cause contraction in smooth muscles, even though the internal physical arrangement of smooth muscle cell fibers is entirely different.

Each vital organ of the body has a very distinct function. The cells of each organ know their specific responsibility in that organ. The smooth muscle cells of each organ are no different. They differ in many ways from organ to organ: physical dimensions, organization into bundles or sheets, response to different types of stimuli, characteristics of innervation, and function. Yet for the sake of simplicity, smooth muscle cells can generally be divided into two major types. Examples of these two types are:

Multi-Unit Smooth Muscle Cell

Some examples of this type of smooth muscle cell are the ciliary muscle of the eye, the iris of the eye and the pilorector muscles (these muscles cause hairs to stand when stimulated by the sympathetic nervous). The most important characteristic of multi-unit smooth muscle cells is each cell can contract independently from the others, and their control is exerted mainly by nerve signals. They seldom exhibit spontaneous contractions. We will talk about these in the chapter about the eyes.

Unitary Smooth Muscle Cell

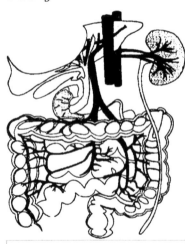

Smooth muscle like that in the digestive tract is involuntary.

Examples of this type of cells include the cells of the intestines, bile ducts, uterus, arteries, lymph veins and other tubes and blood vessels. These smooth muscle cells are usually aggregated into sheets or bundles and their membranes are adherent to one another at multiple points so, force generated in one muscle cell can be transmitted to the next. These smooth cells are used to move fluids or substances through the body. The smooth muscle in the blood vessels also controls blood pressure.

Unlike most skeletal muscles that contract and relax rapidly, most smooth muscle contractions are prolonged tonic contractions, sometimes lasting hours or even days. Therefore, it is to be expected that both the physical and the chemical characteristics of smooth muscle versus skeletal muscle contractions would differ.

Remember, smooth muscle cells contain both actin and myosin filaments, having chemical characteristics similar to those of the actin and myosin filaments in the skeletal muscle cells.

Inside the smooth muscle cell the cycle of the attachment of the myosin to the actin then release from the actin and reattachment is much, much slower than in the skeletal muscle cell. In fact, it is as little as 1/10 to 1/300 the frequency of the skeletal muscle. The energy required to sustain smooth muscle contraction is also only 1/10 to 1/300 as much. This economy of energy utilization by smooth muscle cells is extremely important to the overall energy economy to the body because organs, such as the intestines, urinary bladder, gall bladder and other viscera must maintain tonic muscle contraction almost indefinitely.

A typical smooth muscle cell begins to contract 50–100 milliseconds after it is excited. It reaches full contraction about ½ second later, and then declines in contractile force in another 1 to 2 seconds, giving a total contraction time of 1 to 3 seconds. This is about 30 times as long as a single contraction of an average skeletal muscle. The maximum force of the contraction of smooth muscle is often 50% greater than the skeletal muscle.

Another noteworthy difference is the skeletal muscle has a useful distance of contraction of only about one quarter to one third its stretch length, whereas smooth muscle cells can often contract more than two thirds its stretched length. This allows smooth muscles to perform especially important functions as they change their lumen diameters from very large down to almost zero.

Although skeletal muscle cells are activated exclusively by the nervous system, smooth muscle cells can be stimulated to contract by multiple types of signals: by nervous signals, hormonal stimulation, stretching of the muscle and in several other ways. The principal reason for the difference is smooth muscle cells are able to communicate in several different ways. For instance, when the gut is overfilled by intestinal contents, a local automatic contraction often sets up a peristaltic wave that moves the contents away from the overfilled intestine.

Anyone who has had the experience of rebounding the first thing in the morning will testify that rebounding has an amazing effect on the smooth muscles of digestion. The first experience usually happens within the first few minutes. Fluid begins to accumulate in the kidneys and the smooth muscle cells of the kidneys begin to send messages to the consciousness that a trip to the bathroom is immediately necessary. Approximately ten minutes into rebounding the same type of message is received from the cells of the colon. Again, rebounding has to be postponed.

These are two messages we are readily able to read. We may be unaware of the other messages sent to the rest of the digestive system during rebounding, but several messages you can count on.

"Smooth muscle cells, it is your responsibility of becoming stronger, more efficient, better coordinated and healthier."

Those messages are delivered every time you land on the rebounder because of the increased G-Force effect. As with every other cell of your body, the smooth muscle cells will automatically make the necessary adjustments to your newfound external and internal environmental stimulation.

Bone Density is a Function of Cells

Do me a favor. Go to any health club or athletic department and ask the experts employed there to show you the exercises they use to strengthen the skeleton. You know, that is the structure inside the body to which all of the voluntary muscles are connected. You will catch them by surprise. They will stutter and stammer and then they will eventually show you several machines. Ask them to show you the machine that is designed to strengthen your bones. They will not be able to because it is not there. The health clubs and athletic directors have overlooked the importance of skeletal strength. We are about to overcome that oversight.

Bone is composed of a tough organic matrix that is greatly strengthened by deposits of calcium salts. The average compact bone contains by weight about 30% matrix and 70% salts. The organic matrix of bone is 90–95% collagen fibers, and the remainder is a gelatinous material called ground substance. The collagen fibers extend primarily along the lines of tensional force. These fibers give bone its powerful tensile strength. Each collagen fiber of compact bone is repeated about every 640 angstroms along its length. The segments of adjacent collagen fibers overlap one another. The crystals also overlap, like bricks in a brick wall.

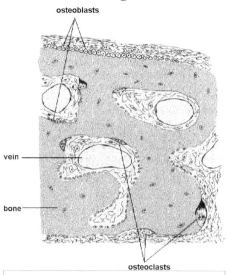

This cross section of a bone shows the osteoid or bone tissue magnified.

The coalition fibers of bone, like those of tendons, have great tensile strength. The calcium salts which are similar in physical properties to marble, have great compression strength. This strength, plus the strength of bonds between the collagen fibers and the crystals make the bone a structure that has both extreme tensile and compression strength. Thus, bones are constructed in the same way reinforced concrete is constructed. The steel of reinforced concrete provides the tensile strength, while the cement, sand and rock provide the compression strength. The compression strength of bone is greater than the best reinforced concrete, and the tensile strength approaches that of reinforced concrete.

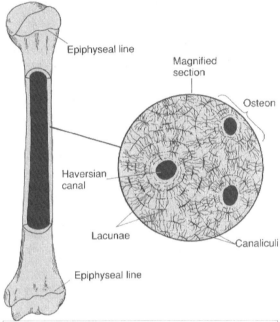

One the outside, bone tissue seems dead and calcific, but bone tissue is actually a very dynamic living tissue which is constantly restructuring itself to compensate for micro fissures in the calcium salts.

But who or what is responsible for building the magnificent bone? The blueprint of the entire skeleton is indelibly recorded in every one of the cells of the body. The initial stage in bone production is the secretion of collagen molecules by bone cells called osteoblasts. The resultant tissue becomes osteoid, a collagen like material which differs from cartilage in that calcium salts will soon precipitate in it. As the osteoid is formed, some of the osteoblasts become entrapped in the osteoid and then are called osteocytes.

Within a few days after the osteoid is formed calcium salts begin to precipitate on the surfaces of the collagen fibers. The precipitate first appear at intervals along each collagen fiber, forming minute nidi that rapidly multiply and grow over a period of days and weeks into the finished product.

Remodeling of Bone

Bone is continually being deposited by osteoblasts and is continually being absorbed where osteoclasts are active. Osteoblasts are found on the outer surface of the bones and in the bone cavities. A small amount of osteoblastic activity occurs continually in all living bones so, at least some new bone is being formed constantly.

Absorption of Bone and the Osteoclasts

Bone is also being continually absorbed in the presence of osteoclasts. Normally, except in growing bones, the rates of bone deposit and absorption are equal to each other so, the total mass of bone remains constant. Osteoclasts usually exist in small but concentrated masses, and once a mass of osteoclasts begin to develop, it usually eats away at the bone for about three weeks, eating out a tunnel that ranges in diameter from 0.2 to 1 millimeters and is several millimeters long. At the end of this time, the osteoclasts disappear and the tunnel is invaded by osteoblasts; then new bone begins to develop. Bone deposition then continues for several months, the new bone is laid down in successive layers of concentric circles on the inner surfaces of the cavity until the tunnel is filled. Deposition of new bone ceases when the bone begins to encroach on the blood vessels supplying the area. It appears that bone cells are very intelligent. They know when to tear down and when to build up the bones.

The continual deposition and absorption of bone has a number of important functions. First, bone ordinarily adjusts its strength in proportion to the degree of bone stress. Consequently, bones thicken when subjected to heavy loads. Second, even the shape of the bone can be rearranged for proper support of mechanical forces by deposition and absorption of bone in accordance with stress patterns. Third, because old bone becomes relatively brittle and weak, new organic matrix is needed as the old organic matrix degenerates. In this manner the toughness of bone is maintained.

The bones of children, in whom the rates of deposition and absorption are rapid, show little brittleness in comparison with the bones of old age, at which time the rates of deposition and absorption are slow.

> "...she [nurse practioner] couldn't believe my age. She said, 'you have the bones of a 17 year old!' The reading was done with a Sahara Clinical Bone Sonometer and measured a T-score of 2.8. Pretty amazing for someone my age. I'm sure that this test was a result of my exercise on a rebounder, my eating habits and good mental health. Thank you Al for all your research and dedication to this form of exercise. It works wonders if you work at it."
>
> email from: Sue Tripp

Bone is deposited in proportion to the compression load the bone must carry. The bones of athletes become considerably heavier than those of non-athletes. Also, if a person has one leg in a cast and uses crutches to get around but continues to walk on the opposite leg, the bone of the leg in the cast becomes thin and as much as 30% decalcified within a few weeks, whereas the opposite bone remains thick and normally calcified. Therefore, continual physical stress stimulates osteoblastic deposition and calcification of bones. Doctors often use walking casts to make sure the injured leg remains properly calcified.

The bodies of our astronauts found that strong bones are not necessary in a zero gravity environment so, the osteocytes (bone cells) became osteoclasts and began to dissolve bone mineral from the bones.

Increasing the G-Force, by rebounding, sends a message to the bone cells telling them the entire skeletal system needs to be mineralized, dense and strong. *This reduces the chance of or even reverses the effects of osteoporosis.* The bone cells are intelligent enough to recognize an increased G-Force demands stronger bones and they simply set about producing a stronger skeleton.

Chapter Eleven

The Lymphatic System

The Internal Environment is Affected by Gravity

So far we have been talking about the various types of cells, their differences and their similarities. We have also presented ways certain cells react to rebound exercise. One thing we cannot overlook is how rebound exercise affects the total environment of the cells. Now if we were studying the human body from the point of view of most exercise physiologists, we would look at the muscles first, then how they move the skeleton. We would look at the cardiovascular system from the heart first and then how the blood carries oxygen and nutrients to the muscles and skeleton.

Since we are introducing rebounding as a cellular exercise, we need to look at the whole body from the cell's point of view. I have heard experts describe the cells as a "bag of fluid with some things in

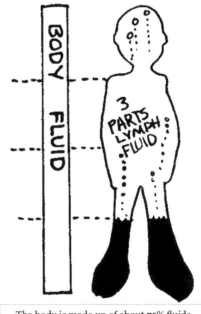

The body is made up of about 75% fluids.

87

it." From the perspective of the cell, "the body is a bag of fluid with some things in it."

All cells live in water—an internal ocean. About 60% of the adult human body is fluid. And depending on where the water is found it is called by various names. If the water is found inside the blood stream it is called plasma. If it is found inside the tissue spaces, muscles, etc. it is called interstitial fluid or extracellular fluid. Water inside the cells is named intercellular fluid, and water captured by the lymphatic system is called lymph fluid. There is also cerebral spinal fluid surrounding the brain and pleural fluid surrounding the lungs. But, except for slight differences in content, it is all water. This clear fluid surrounds all of the internal cells of the body and is in constant motion throughout the body. It is rapidly transporting ions, hormones and nutrients needed by the cells for maintenance of cellular life. The extracellular fluid also washes each of the trillions of cells removing metabolic trash from around the cells. Cells are capable of living, growing and performing their special functions so long as the proper concentrations of oxygen, glucose, different ions, amino acids, fatty substances and other constituents are available in this internal environment.

Homeostasis means the maintenance of static or constant conditions in the internal environment. The maintenance of a relatively constant volume and stable composition of the body fluids is essential for homeostasis. Essentially all of the cells of the organs and tissues of the body perform functions that help to maintain these constant conditions. For instance, the cells of the lungs provide oxygen to the extracellular fluid to replenish continually the oxygen that is being used by the cells, the cells of the kidneys maintain constant ion concentrations and the cells of the gastrointestinal system provide nutrients.

The total body fluid volume and the total amounts of solutes as well as their concentrations are relatively constant during normal conditions, as required for homeostasis. This constancy is remarkable because there is continuous exchange of fluid and solutes with the external environment as well as within the different compartments of the body. For example, there is a highly variable fluid intake that must be carefully matched by equal output from the body to prevent body fluid volumes from increasing or decreasing.

Water is added to the body by ingesting in the form of liquids or water in the food and by the oxidation of carbohydrates. This provides about 2.3 liters/day. Body water is lost by sweating and breathing or through feces and urine. Prolonged exercise can increase the water loss by as much as three times.

Contrary to popular belief the fluid that surrounds the cells of the body is not blood. You see, blood is found only in the cardiovascular system. The 25 trillion red blood cells in the circulatory system traverse the entire circuit an average of once each minute when the body is at rest and as many as six times a minute when the body is extremely active. Their responsibilities are to transport oxygen from the lungs to the capillaries in the tissues and carbon dioxide from the capillaries in the tissues back to the lungs. The body's five to eight pints of blood can only be found in the heart, the arteries, the capillaries and the veins. It is a closed circuit system. The red blood cells never leave this system. The tubes that take blood away from the heart are arteries. They have smooth muscles in their lining which control blood pressure. The tubes that return the blood to the heart are veins.

In the lower extremities of the body the veins are filled with one-way valves forcing the blood always upward towards the heart. If it weren't for valves in the veins, the hydrostatic pressure would cause the venous pressure in the feet always to be about +90 mm Hg in a standing adult. Every time one moves the legs or rebounds, one tightens the muscles and compresses the veins either in the muscles or adjacent to them, and this squeezes the blood out of the veins. The valves in the veins are arranged so, the direction of blood flow can be only toward the heart. Every time a person rebounds, moves the legs or even tenses the muscles, a certain amount of blood is propelled toward the heart and the pressure in the veins is lowered. This pumping system is known as the "venous pump" or "muscle pump" and it is efficient enough that under ordinary circumstances, the venous pressure in the feet of a rebounding adult remains close to or less than 25 mm Hg.

If a human being stands perfectly still, the venous pump does not work, and the venous pressures in the lower part of the leg will rise to the full hydrostatic value of 90 mm Hg in about 30 seconds. The pressures in the capillaries also increase greatly, causing fluid to leak from the circulatory system into the tissue spaces. As a result, the legs swell and the blood volume can be lost from the circulatory system, resulting in fainting.

Muscular contractions, body movements and especially movements of the legs assist in pumping the blood back to the heart. This is why the gentle up and down motion of *rebound exercise improves blood circulation dramatically and reduces high blood pressure.*

Capillaries, the smallest tubes of this amazing circulatory system are so small that the red blood cells have to travel through them in single file. They are sieve-like, with holes so small the red blood cells cannot escape from the cardiovascular system through the small holes, but large enough so the plasma (water) full of nutrients and oxygen can readily flow through the holes and into the area around the cells in the tissue spaces. This happens at the arteriole end of the capillaries. At the venule end of capillaries some of the waste products of cellular metabolism in the interstitial tissues slide through the small holes into the blood stream to be taken to the lungs—where the carbon dioxide is removed from the blood and the kidneys—where other metabolic end products are removed from the blood.

Besides red blood cells, white blood cells, oxygen and nutrients, the blood also circulates various protein molecules. The three we need to know about are the albumin, the globulins and the fibrinogens. That is because these three are big enough to cause problems with the osmotic pressure in the tissue spaces surrounding the cells. The more concentrated the plasma proteins are the more they affect the interstitial fluid pressure. Because of their difference in size about 80% of the total pressure difference of the plasma results from the albumin. About 20% are from the globulins, and almost none from the fibrinogens. Therefore, from the point of view of capillary dynamics, it is mainly albumin that is important.

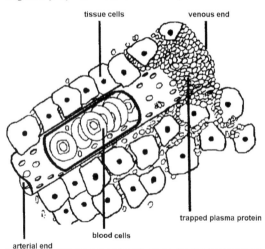

tissue cells   venous end

trapped plasma protein

blood cells

arterial end

Nutrient rich fluid filters out of the arterial end of the capillaries and carries oxygen and nutrients to the cells of the body.

Now that the different factors affecting fluid movement through the capillary membrane have been discussed, it is possible to put all these together to see how normal capillaries maintain normal fluid volume distribution between the plasma and the interstitial fluid.

The average capillary pressure at the arterial ends of the capillaries is 15–25 mm Hg greater than at the venous ends. Because of this difference, fluid filters out of the capillaries at the arterial ends carrying with it oxygen, nutrients and even some plasma proteins. However some of the plasma proteins are so big they cannot fit through the small holes in the capillary walls until the next heart beat. The increased blood pressure at the moment of the heart beat pushes the plasma protein through the small capillary hole into the interstitial fluid where it floats around the outside of the cells. Then the interstitial fluid gradually moves toward the venous end of the capillary where nine tenths of the fluid is sucked back into the blood stream.

Some of the plasma molecules that just barely made it through the capillary wall at the arterial end are now at the venous end. This time there is no pressure pushing the large plasma molecules back into the capillary so, they just begin to sit on the holes of the capillary like plugs in bathtubs. This condition is known as trapped plasma protein. It is a normal condition that happens all over the body. It causes discomfort, itching and pain. If there were no way to correct the condition, death would occur in just a few hours. But the Creator of this body knew the proteins would constantly leak out of the arterial end of the capillaries and would not be able to return back to the blood stream through the venous end. And that is why we have the lymphatic system.

The Lymphatic System

We really do not hear very much about this secondary circulatory system of the body. But regardless of whether you are male or female, young or old, black or white, athlete or couch potato, you have one. If you are like most people you don't even know where your lymph pump is. You know where your blood pump is. You put your hand over it every time you pledge allegiance to the flag. You also know what happens to you when your heart stops beating, but do you know what happens to you if your lymph pump stops working? The following will attempt to give the answer.

> "I've been rebounding for some time now. My initial motivation was lymphatic health. I have found that I can rebound every day (week days) without any signs of over-training. I have tried running on that schedule but developed ankle and knee pain, so I feel rebounding is better for that style of training. I use a 15 minute rebound session to warm up for yoga and weight lifting."
>
> Josh Blacksher

"The lymphatic system represents an accessory route by which fluid can flow from the interstitial spaces into the blood." *Medical Physiology*, A. C. Guyton

The above paragraph deserves rereading. So, I will stop writing for just a moment while you read it again. . . . .

It is also a paragraph that should be memorized by all medical personnel. My personal experience reveals very few people, even in the medical profession, have ever read that paragraph let alone understand its significance. And thus really don't understand the value of the lymphatic system to the health of the body.

The easiest way to explain the lymphatic system is the way a plumber would explain the plumbing inside your house. Almost all tissues of the body have lymphatic channels that drain excess fluid directly from the interstitial spaces. These channels or tubes start in

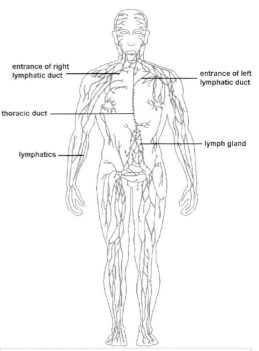

The lymph system is a secondary circulatory system which disposes of metabolic waste. If your lymph system stopped for one day, you would die.

the toes and fingertips and other extremities of the body at lymphatic terminals and connect together in an upside down tree-like fashion until they converge into the thoracic duct, a tube that is approximately as big around as your thumb. The thoracic duct starts just above your navel, and continues vertically between your lungs and finally connects to your blood stream at the vena cava area, just under your collarbone.

Each lymphatic capillary starts at the uniquely designed lymphatic terminal. The lymphatic terminals are never more than two or three cells away from the capillaries of the cardiovascular system.

The terminal functions like a vacuum cleaning nozzle. The cells of the lymphatic terminal are attached by anchoring filaments to the surrounding connective tissue. At the junctions of adjacent

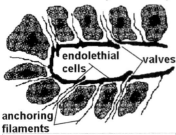

The lymph terminal sucks interstitial fluid and suspended particles from between cells and transports them to the part of the body where they can be either used or disposed of appropriately.

cells, the edge of one cell usually overlaps the edge of the adjacent cell in such a way that the overlapping edge is free to flap inward, thus forming a minute valve that opens to the interior of the lymphatic terminal. Interstitial fluid, along with its suspended particles, is sucked through the open valve and follows directly into the terminal. But this fluid has difficulty leaving the terminal once it has entered because any back flow will close the flap valve. The

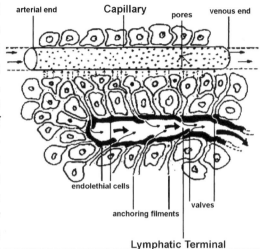

Oversized proteins and ions often leave the circulatory system via pores in the capillaries. It is then the job of the lymphatic system to keep those particles from remaining in between the cells.

only way out is up through the lymph veins.

One-way valves exist in all lymph channels. In the large lymphatics, valves exist every few millimeters. In the smaller lymphatics, much closer than this.

Most of the fluid filtering from the arterial capillaries flows among the cells and is finally reabsorbed back into the venous ends of the blood capillaries; but on the average, probably about one tenth of the fluid enters the lymphatic capillaries instead and returns to the blood through the lymphatic system rather than through the venous capillaries. The total quantity of this lymph is normally only 2 to 3 liters each day.

The minute quantity of fluid that returns to the circulation by way of the lymphatics is extremely important because substances of high molecular weight, such as proteins, cannot be reabsorbed in any other way. Yet they can enter the lymphatic capillaries almost unimpeded because the cells that make up the lymphatic terminal overlap each other and can be moved aside by the fluid pressure created by the suction of the lymphatic system. The vacuuming up of excess interstitial fluid and large particulate matter (including the trapped plasma protein and even bacteria) begins at the millions of lymphatic terminals. The endothelial cells that make up the walls of the terminals are connected to the surrounding tissues by means of their anchoring filaments. So, each time excess fluid enters the tissue and causes the tissue to swell, the anchoring filaments pull the lymphatic capillaries open and fluid flows into the terminal. Then when the tissue is compressed, the pressure inside the terminal increases and causes the overlapping edges of the endothelial cells to close like valves

The lymphatic system is sometimes called the vacuum cleaning system of the body. It is a scavenger system that removes excess fluid, protein molecules, debris and other matter from the tissue spaces.

When fluid enters the terminal, lymphatic capillaries and movement of the tissue propels the lymph forward through the lymphatic system. It eventually empties back into circulation. In this way, any time any free fluid accumulates in the tissues, it is simply pumped away as a consequence of tissue movement. When the amount of fluid leaking from the blood capillaries is slight, which is true for most tissues as research evidence suggests, motion of the tissues and lymphatic capillaries can actually pump a slight intermittent negative pressure that gives an average negativity in the loose tissues.

It has been previously thought that the different tissues of the body are held in place entirely by connective tissue fibers. However, at many places in the body connective tissue fibers are absent. This occurs particularly at points where tissues slide over one another, such as the skin sliding over the back of the hand or over the face. Yet even at these places, the negative interstitial fluid pressure holds the tissues together, creating a partial vacuum by the lymphatic system. When the tissues loose their negative pressure, fluid, metabolic trash, bacteria and excess plasma proteins all accumulate in the spaces and the very unhealthy condition known as edema occurs.

When a larger lymph vessel becomes stretched with fluid, the smooth muscle in the wall of the vessel automatically contracts. So, each segment of the lymph vessel between successive valves functions as a separate automatic pump. The filling of a segment causes it to contract. The fluid is then pumped through the valve into the next lymphatic segment. This fills the subsequent segment, and a few seconds later it too contracts. This continues until the fluid is eventually emptied into the thoracic duct.

Now long before the lymph fluid arrives at the thoracic duct, it filters through one of thousands of lymph nodes strategically located throughout the body. The node is a combination of enemy destruction and army production site. As lymph passes through the lymph node, it is met with hundreds of macrophages, white blood cells, that ingest and digest the large particulate matter and bacteria. They steal the genetic code of the bacteria and prepare an army of white blood cells ready to fight that particular invader the next time it shows up inside the body.

In addition to the pumping caused by the contraction of the lymph vessel walls, external factors that intermittently compress the lymph vessel can also cause pumping. The movement of the surrounding muscles of the body creates intermittent pressure on the lymphatics and assists in the pumping. Movement of body parts such as the swinging of the arms and legs enhances lymph movement inside the vessels. Because the lymph vessels are many times right next to the arteries of the blood stream, pulsations of the arteries create enough pressure to cause lymph to move. Compression of the tissues by objects outside the body such as sitting on a chair, leaning against a wall, simply scratching an itch or rubbing a painful area will increase the pumping action.

Now that we have been exposed to how the lymphatic system actually moves fluid, it is easier to understand that the lymphatic pump becomes very active during rebound exercise, often increasing lymph flow 10–50 fold.

While rebounding, the accelerated upward movement of the body closes the lymph valves forcing all of the lymph fluid upward. At the top of the bounce, the valves open allowing the fluid to move to the next chamber. At the bottom of the bounce the valves slam shut so, the lymph fluid cannot move backwards. Is it necessary to bounce high? No. Your feet don't even have to leave the surface of the mat. This simple up and down modulation is known as the health bounce because this is all that is necessary to turn on the internal vacuum cleaner, the lymphatic system. Four minutes of the simple health bounce will cause the lymphatic system to circulate at least once. If you then dismount the rebounder you will feel a tingling sensation all over your body. All of your cells are sending messages of rejoicing because of their excitingly clean environment.

Chapter Twelve

Improving Body Balance

Body Balance

People usually know in advance if they are able to run up the stairs two at a time or if it is best to hold on to the banister and take it slowly one step at a time. Body balance is a dynamic phenomenon. At its very best, it takes the instantaneous coordination of the vestibular system, the reticular and vestibular nuclei of the brain stem, the antigravity muscles, the proprioceptors and the clear focus of both eyes.

The Vestibular System or The Inner Ear

The vestibule is the organ that is plugged directly into the Earth's gravitation. It is used to detect sensations of equilibrium, stabilization of the head and its own direct relation to the gravitational pull of the earth.

The vestibule is composed of a system of bony tubes and chambers in the temporal bone on each side of the head. This is often called the osseous (bony) labyrinth. Within this is a system of membranous tubes and chambers called the membranous labyrinth. The membranous labyrinth is the functional part of the apparatus. It is composed mainly of the cochlea, three semicircular ducts and two large chambers known as the utricle and the saccule. The cochlea is the major sensory area for hearing and has nothing to do with equilibrium. However, the semicircular ducts, the utricle and the saccule are integral parts of the equilibrium mechanism.

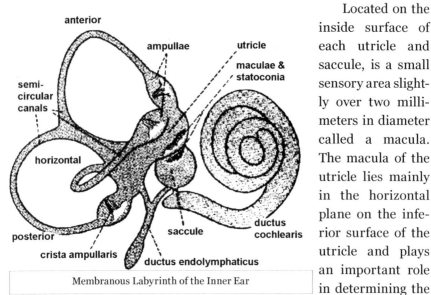

anterior

ampullae

utricle

maculae &
statoconia

semi-
circular
canals

horizontal

posterior

crista ampullaris

saccule

ductus endolymphaticus

ductus
cochlearis

Membranous Labyrinth of the Inner Ear

Located on the inside surface of each utricle and saccule, is a small sensory area slightly over two millimeters in diameter called a macula. The macula of the utricle lies mainly in the horizontal plane on the inferior surface of the utricle and plays an important role in determining the orientation of the head with respect to the direction of the gravitational force when a person is upright. On the other hand, the macula of the saccule is located mainly in a vertical plane and, therefore, is important in equilibrium when a person is lying down.

Each macula is covered by a gelatinous layer in which many small calcium carbonate crystals, called statoconia, are imbedded. Also in the macula are thousands of hair cells. These project up in to the gelatinous layer.

The statoconia have a specific gravity of two to three times as great as the specific gravity of the surrounding fluid and tissues. Therefore, the weight of the statoconia will bend the cilia in the direction of the gravitational pull.

Directional Sensitivity of the Hair Cells

Each hair cell has 50–70 small cilia called sterocilia, plus one large cilium, the kinocilium. The kinocilium is located always to one side, and the sterocilia become progressively shorter toward the other side of the cell. Minute filamentous attachments, almost invisible even to the electron microscope, connect the tip of each stereocilium to the next longer stereocilium and finally to the kinocilium. Because of these attachments when the sterocilia and the kinocilium bend in the direction of the kinocilium, the filamentous attachments tug one after the other on the sterocilia pulling them in the outward direction of the cell body. This opens several hundred channels in each cilium membrane allowing hundreds of positive ions to pour into the cell from the surrounding endoplasmic fluid. This results in depolarization. Conversely, bending the opposite direction reduces the tension on the attachments and this closes the ion channels, thus causing hyper polarization.

Under normal resting conditions, the nerve fibers leading from the hair cells transmit continuous nerve impulses at rates of 100 per second. When the cilia are bent toward the kinocilium, the impulse traffic can increase to several hundred per second. Bending the head in the opposite direction so, the cilia are bent the opposite direction decreases the impulse traffic, often turning it off completely.

In each macula, the different hair cells are oriented in different directions so, some of them are stimulated when the head bends forward, some when it bends backward, others when it bends to one side. Different patterns of excitation occur in the nerve fibers from the macula for each position of the head. It is this pattern that appraises the brain of the head's orientation.

The vestibular system functions extremely effectively for maintaining equilibrium when the head is in the near-vertical position. A normal person can determine as little as a half degree of malequilibrium when the body leans from the precise upright position.

Gymnasts, ice skaters, ballerinas, wrestlers, tennis players and virtually all other active athletes have a much keener sense of equilibrium because through their sport activity they have had to hone their balance through vestibular stimulation. On the other hand, those who do not have a keen sense of balance are babies, senior citizens, invalids and astronauts.

Although there are many ways to stimulate the vestibular system, the most efficient way is to jump on a rebounder. Approximately 100 times a minute the vestibular system is challenged to identify the exact position of the head in the gravitational environment.

Test Your Balance

Stand on the floor next to the rebounder barefoot with your eyes closed. Become aware you are moving back and forth. Recognize you have to rely on your toes and the muscles in your legs and abdomen to maintain your balance.

Now, open your eyes and step into the middle of the rebounder. Close your eyes and begin a gentle up and down bounce and continue for about thirty seconds.

Stop. Step off the rebounder and stand on the floor with your eyes closed. This time you will notice you are very stable—almost as if you have planted your feet in concrete up to your knees.

This is because rebounding stimulates your vestibular system. This is accumulative. As you rebound you will become more aware of the development of your increased balance, which you will be able to take with you to all of your other activities. Stumbling and being clumsy will be things of the past.

The Brain Stem

A part of the body we seldom talk about but depend upon from moment to moment is the brain stem. It is an extension of the spinal cord upward into the cranial cavity. The brain stem provides many special control functions that do not take the conscious thought processes of the brain such as breathing, pumping blood and many other involuntary body functions.

When learning a skill, it takes conscious awareness of the brain to accomplish a particular movement for the first few times. A baby learns how to walk and a child learns how to ride a bicycle this way. For a sixteen year old learning to master the art of driving he must actively engage his brain to turn the practices into skills. However, the thought processes of the brain no longer control the smooth body movements of a tennis player, baseball player, wrestler or gymnast. These learned actions are controlled by the brain stem.

The neurological messages from the vestibular system are sent to the brain stem which in turn sends the necessary body righting messages to the antigravity muscles. These antigravity muscles are the muscles of the vertebral column and the extensor muscles of the limbs. Thus standard gravity opposing actions like standing, walking and sitting take very little cognitive thought. We are able to sit in a movie completely unaware of where our body parts are. Or we carry on an aggressive conversation as we walk, ambivalent to the thousands of neurological messages being sent by the brain stem to ensure we do not fall all over our feet.

While we stand, walk or run, the brain stem receives exacting messages from the proprioceptors in the joints telling how much the joints are bent. The foot pads send messages telling how much weight is on the front of the foot or on the heel and if the weight is equally distributed when walking or standing. This information is analyzed and immediate decisions are made by the brain stem so the brain does not have to be bothered by well practiced functions.

The brain stem contains motor and sensory nuclei that perform motor and sensory functions for the face and head regions. In another sense the brain stem is its own master, because it provides many special control functions such as:

- Control of respiration
- Control of cardiovascular system
- Control of gastrointestinal functions
- Control of many involuntary functions and movements of the body
- Control of equilibrium
- Control of eye movement

In its role of controlling equilibrium, the brain stem is responsible for sending two types of messages to the antigravity muscles. The two sets of messages work antagonistically to each other. One group of messages is sent exciting the antigravity muscles to rigidity. The other group of messages are sent to the same group of muscles to inhibit them from opposing gravity.

The ability of the antigravity muscles to receive the two sets of opposing messages makes it possible for us to participate in simple activities such as sitting, walking, jogging, running, dancing, wrestling and gymnastics. When we participate in the above activities, the neurological messages are sent back and forth between the brain stem and the antigravity muscles so the muscles relax and contract automatically.

Despite the automaticity of these actions, the brain can interact with the brain stem at any time to further hone the balancing mechanisms of the human body. This is necessary when a baseball player is trying to improve his pitch or a golfer is concentrating on improving his swing. It also helps the dancer readjust when she stumbles and falls attempting new dance steps. When a child is learning how to ride a bicycle, the brain tells the brain stem how to react in order to maintain balance. After the skills are learned, the brain stem takes over and receives very little assistance from the brain.

Many times when we attend a health and fitness show as we introduce rebound exercise to the general public, we hear this statement, "I could never bounce on that. I would fall off." The person making that statement was probably in tune with his brain stem. He knew he had not stimulated his brain stem sufficiently to feel comfortable bouncing up and down on a rebounder. This is because he probably trains by walking. Walking does not provide the vertical stimulation to the brain stem necessary to provide confidence in the ability to rebound.

For this reason, we produce balance bars that can be attached to two of the legs of a rebounder. These bars provide support for those who are unsure of their balance. Placing a rebounder next to a wall or a doorframe will also provide stability. We do however believe that the need for stability assistance is only temporary, because rebounding stimulates and strengthens the vestibular system, the functions of the brain stem and all antigravity muscles. Very often a person who orders a stabilizing bar finds they are able to wean themselves from its use. Their new found balance and coordination can then be used in such activities as climbing or descending stairs or even walking without stumbling.

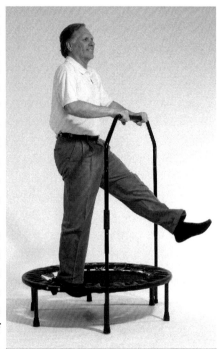

Through experience, we have found rebounding improves normal movements of the body, enhances equilibrium and even stimulates better eye movement. This is one half of all of the responsibilities of the brain stem listed above. Is it possible, by stimulating the brain stem through rebound exercise, other automatic functions such as respira-

Stabilizing bars are valuable for people who want vigorous workouts without worrying about their balance.

tion, cardiovascular and gastrointestinal functions are also improved? If that is the case then rebound exercise is more vital to the health and proper functions of the body than we have previously supposed.

Rebounding and Autism Therapy

Rebounding has also been used in therapy to help autistic people. One mother commented that rebound exercise combined with other exercises helped her child to function more normally while providing him a safe and stimulating exercise. She said in her letter,

"I just wanted to write to you to tell you how wonderful for, and essential to the therapy and daily life of my son with autism spectrum your Rebounder is. Our son is 5'11' at age 15 and about 150 lbs. He is extremely athletic and runs like the wind. This is his extraordinary gift. But ironically, with the autism, he runs out the door and down the street. With the Rebounder he is able to get his exercise without putting his life at the risk of getting hit by a car or being lost. He adores your rebounder and uses it at least an hour a day. He will intermittently get on the rebounder and jump from 3 to 5 minutes. He is very adept at using the Rebounder and would be utterly lost without it.

"With many autistic children there is a real problem with what is called "elopement" which means they run off and do not have a real sense of danger. Sometimes their ability to get exercise is compromised severely as a result. Between the Rebounder and the fact that our son considers doing sit-ups to be recreation, he is very well built, has a sense of his surroundings that he responds to and is much more normal in his bearing and demeanor. The Rebounder is an integral and absolutely necessary part of our son's ongoing therapy." —*Kate Baker*

Thank you Kate for your kind words, and for further showing the flexibility of rebound exercise as a therapeutic tool.

Chapter Thirteen

Enhance your Vision
with Rebound Exercise

As a performing trampolinist, I was approached many times by students, parents and teachers who asked me if I knew why ophthalmologists recommended bouncing on a trampoline to assist young children in their ability to see more clearly. Since I traveled all over the United States as a trampolinist and had heard this question in many different places, it was obvious this was not just a local query. At that time when asked, my answer was simply, "I do not know." In fact, I thought it was very strange that anybody involved in optometry would ever suggest bouncing on a trampoline as therapy. It was not until I got involved in my own research about rebound exercise that I could identify the correlation between jumping on a trampoline and better vision.

Eyesight is a Gift

In His wisdom, our Benevolent Creator gave us eyesight, a possession we own without request. We didn't ask for it. He gave it to us. It comes with the body as a standard feature. It is good that it's a gift, be-

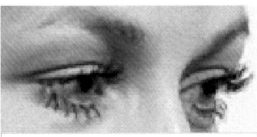

As much as 80% of the information we gather about our environment is collected through the eyes.

cause if we'd never experienced the beauty of seeing, how could we know that eyesight even existed, let alone put in our requisition for it?

For most of us, eyesight comes completely assembled and plugged in ready to use. This is a good thing. We depend on sight so much that experts claim we may use it to gather as much as 80% of the information about our world in which we reside. The only way we really know of its value is by comparing good eyesight to less than perfect eyesight or no eyesight at all.

We depend upon eyesight more than any other sense to supply vital information about our surrounding environment. Some information we gather through sight is about the food we eat, the times and seasons, mortal danger or even knowledge gained through the writings of great authors. Wouldn't it be a great idea to learn more about this marvelous gift so as to be able to use it more effectively?

Eye and head mobility combined with stereoscopic sight (eyesight from two slightly different angles) provide humans with a panoramic view of the world, containing information on depth, distance, dimension and movement. All of this you received when you were born, with no strings attached. It was simply a gift written into the genetic code of each of your cells.

The Gift is not ours Alone

The ability to see is truly a gift, but we are not the only beings who possess it. Even certain single celled creatures that live in the sea have areas called eyespots that are sensitive to light.

Most eyes come in twos—fish, animals, insects and birds—but there are also exceptions, such as eight eyed spiders and one eyed crustaceans.

The design, placement and use of the eyes vary greatly to suit the needs of the owner. The dragonfly, who lives

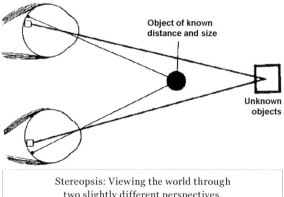

Object of known distance and size

Unknown objects

Stereopsis: Viewing the world through two slightly different perspectives.

on smaller insects, must be able to spot gnats anywhere around it. Maybe that is why it has been provided with eyes which do not move, but look every way at once. In some varieties of dragonfly, each eye has as many as twenty-eight thousand separate hexagonal facets! Each facet sees a tiny part of the whole picture.

The anableps, a tiny tropical fish, feeds on the surface of the water but has to keep an eye partly open for predators below the water. It has bifocal eyes just like bifocal spectacles so, it can focus on things above and below the surface of the water as necessary.

Eagles and owls can spot rabbits and mice thousands of feet below their flight path because their eyes are positioned forward, but the rabbit can see all around without moving its head because its eyes bulge to the side of its head, thus seeing the attacking bird of prey.

The Eye: The Creator's Masterpiece

The eye is one of the Creator's most magnificent masterpieces—elegant in design, efficient in function and intricate in construction. The eye is made up of millions of very intelligent cells. Each cell of the eye is assigned a simple task which is recorded in the DNA and is required to perform that task to perfection. Some cells are charged with special chemicals capable of identifying certain colors. Others must control the intensity of light entering the eye. Some are responsible for refracting light and still other cells are capable of controlling the amount of light entering the eye. Some cells read only that part of the DNA that tells them how to become minute muscle cells while other cells become the outside white surface or the inside dark gray surface of the eyeball.

In the embryo, the retina develops from the optic vesicle, an epithelial out pocketing of the forebrain. This epithelium makes contact with the ectoderm covering the exterior of the head. That is the signal for certain cells to form the lens. At the same time some cells develop into the hollow, round ball. Other adjoining cells become muscle cells in the six muscles strategically located around the outside. These muscles control the direction of each eye. Other cells take on the appearance of a rigid curved transparent window in the front of the eye. The clear cornea, the bulge at the front, lets light rays into the eye and bends or refracts them.

The round case or outside covering, of the eyeball, apart from the transparent cornea at the front, is made of cells, which form tough, white fibrous tissue. We call this the sclera of the eye. The cells of the sclera are nourished by minute blood vessels. When the eye is irritated, say by dust, chlorine or an infection, the blood vessels become enlarged and the "white" of the eye appears pink or bloodshot.

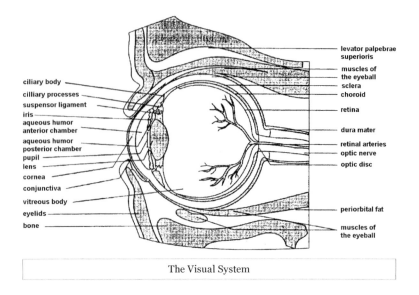

The Visual System

A flat, circular, colored membrane composed of several layers of microscopic muscle cells lies behind the cornea and gives the eyes their characteristic colors. This is called the iris. The iris governs the size of the pupil—a small hole in its center—and regulates the amount of light entering the eye.

Between the cornea and the iris is a small compartment containing a clear fluid, the aqueous humor, which nourishes the cornea, the iris and the lens. Normally the aqueous is supplied by fluid which flows into the eyeball from the lymphatic system into the vitreous humor or the fluid behind the lens and in front of the back of the eye. It then flows past the lens, through the iris and the pupil. It then filters out between the iris and the cornea through the Canal of Schlem.

Clear cells organize themselves near the middle front of the eye into a spherical lens. The crystalline lens, positioned behind the pupil, further refracts the light to focus a sharp image on the retina.

There are six muscles on the outside of each eye through which the eye functions. These are called extrinsic muscles, meaning on the outside of the eye. Four of these muscles attach to the sclera near the front of the eye, one above, one below and one on each side. They extend from near the cornea in front of the eye to the bony structure at the back of the eyeball. They are called recti muscles.

The other two extrinsic muscles circle the eye obliquely, thus acquiring the name oblique muscles. One of these oblique muscles is attached to the sclera at the lower side of the eyeball, the other to the upper side of the

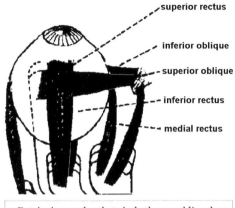

superior rectus

inferior oblique

superior oblique

inferior rectus

medial rectus

Extrinsic muscles that circle the eye obliquely.

eyeball. These muscles are both voluntary and involuntary.

Muscles cannot push. They can only pull. That is why most muscles work in opposing pairs. In the case of the extrinsic muscles of the eye, they work as a team. They are used to turn the eye up and down, from side to side, around and around and even converge on close objects, by crossing the eyes.

Another function of the extrinsic muscles is to assist the eye in focusing on near or far objects. Think for a moment that the eye is like a grape caught in a sling. As tension increases on the recti muscles, the eye would have a tendency to flatten thus helping to accommodate for farsightedness. As the recti muscles relax and the oblique muscles tighten, the eye elongates for up close sight.

The muscle cells inside the eyeball itself, intrinsic muscle cells, are found in two circular structures.

The iris, the colored or pigmented part of the eye, is composed of two types of muscles. These two muscle types govern the size of the opening (the pupil). One of these types is arranged in a circular fashion, while the other extends in a radial manner like the spokes of a wheel.

The ciliary body is shaped somewhat like a flattened ring with a hole the size of the outer edge of the iris. The ciliary muscle cells alter the shape of the lens during the process of accommodation.

The purpose of the iris is to regulate the amount of light entering the eye. If a strong light is flashed in the eye, the circular muscle fibers of the iris, which form a sphincter, contract and thus reduce the size of the pupil. On the other hand, if the light is very dim, the radial involuntary iris muscle cells, which are attached at the outer edge, contract. The opening is pulled outward and thus enlarged. This pupillary enlargement in known as dilation. The pupil also changes size according to whether one is looking at a near object or a distant one. Viewing a near object causes the pupil to become smaller; a far view will cause it to enlarge.

The process of adjustment for near and distant vision (accommodation) is controlled, in part, by manipulating the curvature of the crystalline lens. The lens of the eye, although it resembles a piece of curved glass, differs from glass in that it is not a homogenous material. It consists instead of approximately 2000 thin layers of clear cell tissue. As the light rays pass through each layer they are refracted to a minute degree. The lens of the eye differs from glass in another important way, it's flexible. The lens of a camera, for example, has to be moved backwards or forward until the correct focus is found, the lens of the eye simply changes shape. It becomes thin when one is looking at distant objects and becomes thick when objects of interest are near . A sheath of transparent material called the suspensory ligament supports the lens. The eye adjusts its focus by changing the curvature or thickness of the lens.

The muscle of the ciliary body is similar in layout and function to the radial muscle of the iris. The ciliary muscles work in harmony with the suspensory ligament. When the ciliary muscle cells contract, they remove the tension on the suspensory ligament of the lens causing the ligament to relax. When the ligament is relaxed the elastic lens recoils becoming thicker. Think of the lens as a rubber band that thickens when tension is released. When the ciliary muscle cells relax, the suspensory ligament becomes tense and pulls the lens flat. These actions change the refractive ability of the lens.

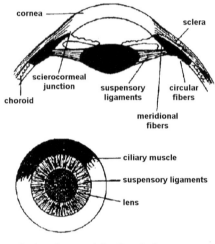

mechanism of accomodation (focusing)

A cross section of the muscles that help the lense to adjust and focus for near and far sight.

When you are focusing on a close up object, a complicated process occurs. As mentioned previously, your ciliary muscles contract thickening your lenses, the circular muscle fibers of the irises contract to decrease the size of the pupils. At the same time the lateral rectus of both eyes (closest to the nose) tighten while the outside lateral rectus relaxes slightly, this causes the eyes to converge on the target object.

By the way, Dr. William Bates, Ophthalmologist, proved in his work that accommodation (focusing for near and far seeing) is not completely dependent on the lens of the eye. Eyes which have had the lens removed due to a cataract operation were able to learn to accommodate for this loss by the action of the rest of the eye muscles.

It is possible to strain any or all of these muscles with unwise, sharp movements such as unaccustomed visual exercises, just as it is possible to strain or sprain the muscles, ligaments and tendons of an arm or ankle. A sprained eye muscle will probably produce no permanent damage, but it is inconvenient and painful just like other sprained muscles.

Protection of the eyeball and All Its Parts

In the embryo, the eye develops as an out pocketing of the brain. The eye is a delicate organ, and the Creator has carefully protected it by means of the following structures:

- The skull bones form the eye orbit (cavity) and serve to protect more than half of the dorsal part of the eyeball.
- The eyelids and eyelashes help protect the eye from dust and floating debris.
- Tears wash away small foreign objects that may enter the eye.
- A sac lined with an epithelial membrane separates the front of the eye from the eyeball proper and aids in the destruction of some of the pathogenic bacteria that may enter from the outside.

Coats of the Eyeball

The eyeball has three separate coats or tunics. The outermost layer is called the sclera and is made of firm tough connective tissue. It is commonly referred to as the white of the eye. The second tunic of the eyeball is the choroid coat. Composed of a delicate network of connective tissue interlaced with many blood vessels, this layer contains much dark brown pigment. The choroid may be compared to the dull black lining of a camera. It prevents incoming light rays from scattering and reflecting off the inner surface of the eye. The innermost coat, called the retina, includes ten layers of nerve cells, including the end organs commonly called the rods and cones.

These are the receptors for the sense of vision. The rods are sensitive to white and black. The cones are sensitive to color. As far as is known, there are three types of cones, each of which is sensitive to red, green or blue. Persons who completely lack cones are totally colorblind; those who lack one type of cone are partially colorblind. Color blindness is an inherited condition and occurs mainly in males.

Pathway of Light Rays

Light rays, which normally travel in straight lines through the air, are refracted or change direction slightly when they enter a denser medium, such as water or glass. The eye uses refraction to focus the light rays that reflect off the world and into the retina. Some light is always necessary for seeing. The human eye cannot perceive images of an object unless light rays carry it. A luminous source, such as a candle, may either send light directly to the eye or the rays may bounce off of it. They can also be reflected by the surface of an object before reaching the eye.

Light rays pass through a series of transparent eye parts. On the way they undergo a process of bending known as refraction. This refraction of light rays makes it possible for light from a very large area to be focused on the retina, where the receptors are located. The following are the transparent refracting parts (or media of the eye) from the outside in.

The cornea is a forward continuation of the outer coat, but it is transparent and colorless, where as the sclera is opaque and white. The cornea is referred to frequently as the "window" of the eye. It bulges forward slightly and is the most important refracting structure. Light first passes through the cornea and the rays are refracted because the cornea is denser than air. This begins the process of focusing an image onto the retina. Since the cornea bends the light rays more than any other part of the eye, it is referred to as the coarse focus.

The aqueous humor, a watery fluid which fills much of the eyeball between the cornea and the lens, helps to maintain the slight forward curve in the cornea.

Control of the amount of light entering the eye is essential to keep the retinal image from being blurred. The combined automatic response of the contraction and expansion of the muscle fibers in the iris determines the amount of light let in through the pupil. This control is particularly important when sharpness of acuity is required by detailed work. For instance, in close-up work such as reading, the pupil shrinks in order to sharpen the focus by limiting the access of light rays to a tiny point.

The crystalline lens is a circular structure made of a flexible rubbery material. The lens has two bulging surfaces. It may be best described as biconvex. During youth, the lens is elastic, and therefore its thickness can be readily adjusted according to the need for near or distance vision.

The vitreous humor is a jelly-like substance that fills the entire space behind the lens and helps to keep the eyeball in its spherical shape.

The retina, the screen on which light rays are projected, is a network of more than 130 million tightly packed cells covering the transparent innermost layer of the eyeball. The nerve fibers are composed of two types of light sensitive receptors, rods and cones.

These two types of cells allow us to exist comfortably in two visual worlds—day and night, light and dark. The information telling how to

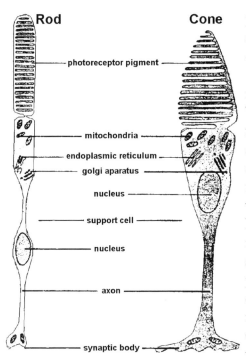

Rod　　　　　**Cone**

- photoreceptor pigment
- mitochondria
- endoplasmic reticulum
- golgi aparatus
- nucleus
- support cell
- nucleus
- axon
- synaptic body

Cones have different sizes of photoreceptors, which allow them to detect the differences in the wavelengths of light, or the pigments. Rods do not detect those fine differences between color, but gauge between lights and darks which is perfect for night vision.

produce rods and cones is also available in the DNA of all cells of the body.

Cells that take on the job of identifying just black and white become the rods. Rods are used for seeing in dim light. Rods respond only to shades of black and white. They contain a chemical, rhodopsin, also known as visual purple. Rhodopsin allows the rods to function only in dim light, where colors are subdued and often lost completely. Bright light bleaches the chemical, reducing the sensitivity of the visual system to light. Consequently, when a person walks into a dark room from a sunny garden he is temporarily "blinded" until the visual purple is formed again.

Cells that take on the responsibility of identifying color based on the length of the light rays, become the cones. A mixture of cones and rods are distributed unevenly in the retina. In the center of the retina, the fovea contains only cones and is used for accurate vision in bright light. The seven million cones are used to examine an object in bright light. They are assisted in this effort by the chemical, iodopsin, which is sensitive to colored light.

The macula lutea is a small yellow spot the size of the head of a pin. It is located at the center of the retinal nerve tissue. In the very center of the macula lutea is a small depression called the fovea centralis. When it is properly focused, the eye receives the sharpest possible picture. This is the true center of sight. This little fovea centralis has a natural oscillating movement of seventy times a second and, unknown to you, moves as a tiny paintbrush over the reflection of the object on which you are focusing. When you focus on a small area of an object, you are using the fovea point. The eye could be likened to a bowl whose sides slant upward or an arena with a small field. The fovea, the dot of perfect vision, is at the bottom of the field arena. This is the only part of the eye that has strong clear vision. It sees a central object, like a rose in a vase, while the surrounding objects are seen secondarily. The secondary vision is called peripheral vision.

This thin, nerve laden screen lining the back of the eye transforms light energy into electrical messages which are transmitted to the brain by the optic nerve. The optic nerve runs from the back of the eye to the visual cortex, (that part of the brain responsible for interpreting vision).

The adaptability of the eye and its sensitivity to colors and contours enables man to perform close and detailed tasks at one moment and scan the clouds on the horizon the next.

Eyes do not actually see. They are perfect color television aerials. As aerials, they are incredible receivers of a myriad of wavelengths of light. When an object is first registered on the retina, it is conveyed by nerve impulses by way of the optic nerve. These wavelengths are transmitted to two "television screens" in the brain located in the back of the head where interpretation occurs. Our ability to see clearly occurs when an accumulation of information is neuro-electrically transferred to the visual cortex of the brain. So, you do not actually see with your eyes. You see with your brain. The visual cortex dwells in total darkness. Instantaneously, the cells of the visual cortex "develop" the images received from the nerve impulses and compare the picture to the information already stored in your memory.

Our Lack of Vision about Vision

The odds are five to one you are reading this book through glasses quite similar to the ones worn by Benjamin Franklin. The frames may be more ornate and better fitted to your face than the wire rims that hung on Franklin's ears and saddled his nose, but the functions and expected results are about the same. Or you may be one of over a hundred million people who wear contact lenses. It is estimated 50% of all adults in the United States wear glasses. About 95% of all adults over forty-five wear glasses. Regardless of your age, once you start wearing glasses you are expected to wear them the rest of your life. You probably have already accepted the concept that when you do change your glasses, you will need stronger lenses.

Naturally, you are under the impression you are wearing glasses because you need them. The odds are, however, four to one the real reason you are wearing glasses is because you do not know it is possible to live quite comfortably without them. All you need to get started is a little knowledge about your magnificent body, incredible eyes, visual talents, rebound exercise and proper nutrition.

Vision is a Talent

Most people use the terms "vision" and "eyesight" interchangeably when there really is a distinct difference. We have already established that eyesight is a gift, the ability to see objects in your environment. When you are born and you open your eyes, you see so, you have eyesight, but you do not have vision. Vision is not a gift. You have to work for it. It is a learned talent or a whole group of talents. It is something that has to be earned.

Immediately after birth you begin to practice focusing your eyes. Soon you are able to follow the finger of the doctor as he checks your ability to see. You continue to practice and gain experience until you recognize the source of your nourishment, which comes not just from eye signals but from other senses as well. You begin to identify "clues," which in turn enhance your vision. The cooing of mother, her smell, the softness of your blankets and the security of your bed. As you pick up on these clues, your vision improves. Soon you will learn that mother always comes to you through the door so, the door becomes a source of love and affection. But the door also separates you from mother so, it becomes an enemy and you begin to cry every time the door closes behind her as she leaves.

Nothing in your environment means anything to you until you have had some form of introduction to it. The wall sockets are only of interest to you because they are there in your environment, until you learn of their danger. Mother pulls you away before you stick a hairpin in the holes. When you are older you learn the on switch of the television doesn't work when mother pulls the plug.

Vision is a talent or learned procedure. It is something you can and should develop throughout your entire life. Think of it this way: just because a person is born with fingers doesn't mean he knows how to play the piano. Playing the piano is a talent and it takes many hours of dedication to master it. Likewise, a person owning eyes does not necessarily have good vision.

The definition, then, of vision is: *The ability to identify your total environment with the least number of clues.* If, for the sake of this discussion, we can accept that definition of vision, then understanding what your "total environment" is will help you to enhance your vision. It could also infer that although Helen Keller did not have the use of her eyes or her ears, she quite possibly had very good vision.

The human body uses primarily vision to analyze and match the seen information against the cumulative experience of the whole organism. Sight helps you in tasks like finding your way to your seat in a darkened theater, trying to understand an esoteric poem or slam dunking a basketball.

In many respects, vision is a learned skill, as complex a process as learning to speak. Speaking is an attempt to share thoughts or visions. Vision is the ability to comprehend how you should function from moment to moment. Vision is also crucial to preparing for the future.

Vision, then, is interplay between sight and all other human senses. Although the eyes play a major roll in vision, it is only part of the whole picture. Nearly 80% of everything we learn comes through our eyes. The other four senses verify what is seen.

Visual deficiencies should not therefore be regarded as fixed, irreversible physical flaws, but as problems correctable through training. Proper training can lead the whole body/mind system to "see" more efficiently. No one should give up and assume that improvement won't come. You have nothing to lose, but the whole world to see.

Eyesight may be defined as merely seeing, but vision involves synthesizing, unifying and understanding what is being seen. Vision is therefore no mere passive event, but a complicated and largely learned process that occurs mainly in the brain. Thus a person's ability to locate, interpret and manipulate physical objects in his field of vision is directly related to his ability to create, think and solve problems.

A round object across the room looks like a white ball until you bite into it. You then taste, smell and feel that it is an onion. You have just enhanced your vision because the next time, you neither have to taste, smell nor feel the onion. You can then identify part of your environment with fewer clues. Vision, then, goes beyond the eyes. It includes the other senses of touch, taste, smell and hearing along with other talents such as balance, coordination, rhythm, timing, kinesthetic awareness and posture.

I See What You Mean

Dr. A.M. Skeffington, the single most important pioneer in the field of visual training, was born in Nebraska at the turn of the century. He was born to a seafaring English father and an intellectual Danish mother who was educated at the "Royal Court School" in Copenhagen.

After going to a theological seminary at Nashota, Wisconsin, Skeffington, a man with an insatiable curiosity and a passion for logic, finally dropped out of school and went west for several years to work. He herded sheep, wrangled cattle, hauled hay and worked on a railroad section gang. Eventually he drifted into the study of optometry. In that calling, he seemed to have found the lifelong challenge he was seeking.

Largely self-educated, he probed the mysteries of human vision. He was the first educational director of the Optometric Extension Program and for forty years thereafter, he was the guiding spirit of this organization. Those who followed and believed in Skeffington have built up his insight and added valuable findings of their own through research, observation and experience with their patients.

Modern optometrists have developed a comprehensive, holistic approach to visual training based on the belief that the visual system leads, coordinates and thus greatly influences all functions of the body and mind. It aims at improving the overall efficiency of the whole person. Their aim is a more harmonious focus on the efficient relationship between vision, posture, muscular coordination and the working of the brain. This is why they measure success not only by improvement in the clarity and sharpness of the eyesight (whether the patient is able at the end to throw away his glasses), but rather by a better general performance—physical and mental—with or without glasses.

Our Visual Experts

As we consider the health of our eyes, it is so important for us to understand our visual experts. Many people get the terms opticians, optometrists, oculists and ophthalmologists mixed up.

An **ophthalmologist** is a medical doctor who specializes in the treatment of eyes. One who has passed an examination by a State Board of Optometry. He is able to provide surgery, medication, therapy and glasses for accidents, injury, birth defects and imperfect vision.

An **optometrist** is not a medical doctor but he has also passed an examination provided by a State Board of Optometry. This gives him authority to measure the extent and character of eye defects. He prescribes corrective lenses, but does not treat pathological conditions.

An **optician** is a skilled technician who grinds and sells optical lenses according to prescription. Like a pharmacist, he prepares and sells medication according to a prescription from a medical doctor.

An **oculist** is a medical doctor who treats the eyes, but he does not have special training in eye care beyond standard medical education.

A **vision therapist** is a vision coach. This person is convinced vision can be improved by some type of environmental change. Vision Therapists come from all types of educational backgrounds. Some are teachers who are concerned about educational handicaps or optometrists interested in improving vision through training lenses or other means.

Each state has different laws regulating licensing procedures for vision therapists. In some states they are not officially recognized, while in other states they are licensed and able to advertise. In my investigation of the licensing procedure, there is nothing demanding an eye specialist to know anything about exercise or nutrition.

Rebound to the Rescue

The first time the term, "Rebound Exercise" was in print was August 1977, when I published *Rebound to Better Health*. But until May of 1979, almost nothing was written about rebound exercise as a form of vision therapy. *The Miracles of Rebound Excercise*, published in 1979, has one chapter on it. *The New Miracles of Rebound Excercise* only refers to it.

The National Institute of Reboundology and Health, Inc. produced its first Vision Therapy kit in 1980 and sold over 10,000 kits in the next two years. A survey of the users of the kit revealed 92% noticed a definite visual improvement. Rebounding has been used for over fifty years by visual therapists in their laboratories and clinics. They report their results as very positive.

G. N. Gettman, O. D., wrote an article entitled, "Use of the Trampoline in the Developmental Visual Guidance" over fifty years ago stating,

"A trampoline, a device for rebound tumbling, has usually been considered gymnastic equipment, and too frequently one of its real values has been overlooked... the trampoline provides opportunities for the acquisition of basic movement control, which is essential to coordination of all the motor skills including vision. Clinical and research studies of rebound tumbling indicate the trampoline can provide experiences that influence a child's academic success. Many authorities recognize a child's freedom to learn and his readiness for new learning experiences is dependent on his freedom and control of movement. This control of movement must come from the visual mechanism because the eyes are the primary steering machinery for all movements. The trampoline contributes more to the organization of visual perception than any other known device..."

Although little was written on the subject, the value of rebounding was common knowledge among eye specialists. Here's what one doctor said after I finished a 2 hour lecture to ophthalmologists on visual enhancement through rebound exercise. After the lecture he shot up out of his seat and exclaimed to the other specialists, "I have been using a small trampoline in my practice for over twenty years now, and this is the first time anyone explained why it works so well." (Lecture given at the Red Lion Hotel just off the Sea Tac Airport near Seattle)

You may ask if the eyes need physical exercise. The answer is "yes." Most of us get our exercise quite simply by using our eyes, much the same way we exercise the rest of our body by simply using it. But, for some people an eye specialist has indicated they have amblyopia or "lazy eye". This simply means one of their eyes has for some reason decided to do most or all of the work, allowing the control muscles of the other eye to become weak through lack of exercise.

The very fact that amblyopia exists is proof enough the cells of the eyes and the muscles of the eyes can be weakened with lack of exercise. Logic tells us exercising them can also strengthen them. Your eyes need the right kind of exercise—cellular exercise. Rebounding is that cellular exercise.

There are those people, including possibly your friends, relatives or even visual experts who will say good nutrition and exercise will not alter the eyeball and the only solution for poor vision is glasses. They will say glasses are designed to accommodate for the eyeball being either too short or too long. They do not give enough credit to the extrinsic muscles, which assist in focusing on near or far objects.

As the recti muscles relax and the oblique muscles tighten, the eye elongates for nearsightedness. Exercise the recti muscles sufficiently and they will adjust for both far and near sightedness. There are at least two ways to strengthen these muscles.

- Practice looking far and near without glasses, and
- Participate in a cellular exercise that strengthens all muscle cells regardless of where they are in the body.

Eyes, as well as the rest of your body, are products of genetics and your environment. For the most part, they change upon demand.

Not everyone who uses rebound techniques will be so successful as to be able to eliminate their need for glasses. Still, virtually everyone who can see will be able to improve their vision to some degree because of the added knowledge, exercise, circulation and stimulation provided by rebounding. It is my feeling that well over 50% of all people who wear glasses today could wean themselves from them if they had the knowledge and the desire to do so. The problem is we really don't know which 50% can really do it. So, the question is simple. What do you have to loose? Or better yet, what do you have to gain?

We know it works. The only question is: Are you one of the 50% of those who are wearing glasses who may not need glasses if given the right opportunity? If you are willing to dedicate some of your time to eliminate your need for glasses, we have an exciting kit for you. Order *Enhance Your Vision with Rebound Exercise*, and start seeing what you have been missing.

Chapter Fourteen

How much Exercise is Enough?

In 1977, I made the statement, "Rebound Exercise is the most efficient, effective form of exercise yet devised by man."

A study by the University of Utah pointed out rebound exercise eliminates seven eighths of the bone jarring skeletal shock experienced by runners who run on a gymnasium floor.

NASA's 1981 study published in the *Journal of Applied Physiology*, stated among other things that rebounding was as much as 68% more efficient than treadmill jogging. What did they mean by "more efficient?"

The Institute of Aerobics Research, of Dallas, Texas produced a study on weight training and rebounding. This study showed that in just twelve weeks, people who rebounded for thirty seconds in between each weight training station (in a circuit weight training system) can expect to increase in strength by as much as 25% over those who did not rebound between stations!

It is little wonder that James White Ph.D., author of *Jump for Joy*, stated, "Rebounding is the closest thing to the Fountain of Youth that science has found."

Still, the biggest question, "How much exercise is enough?" remained unanswered until just recently.

Many exercise experts endorse the Twenty Minute Target Zone Theory, but not for reasons I can completely accept. I have yet to find anyone who can tell me what is magic about twenty minutes. Why not thirty or twelve? Will three minutes do the job if done consistently, say, twice a day? We have reasons to believe so. That is, the number one reason to exercise is for the "health of it."

Now, we recognize there are those who are exercising for the purpose of competing in some sporting event. The majority of us are exercising simply because we want to live longer and be more healthy. Most adults are not interested in running a 10 K even if they were good athletes in high school or college. They simply want to be healthy, have more energy and be efficient at whatever they wish to do.

Twelve years ago, a landmark study was published indicating physical activity is related to reduction in all causes of death and to increased longevity. Now a major new study confirms that a person's physical fitness level is related to a delay in "all-cause mortality". The first study came from Dr. Ralph Paffenbarger's famous research of 16,936 Harvard University alumni over a period of 16 years. The second study is based on data from 13,344 people followed over an average of eight years by Steven Blair at the Institute of Aerobics Research, Dallas, Texas. (Published in the Journal of the American Medical Association, Nov. 3, 1989.)

While the former study asked Harvard alumni about their activities and calculated their weekly caloric expenditure, the new study measured participants' fitness by a maximal treadmill exercise test. We can accept the treadmill exercises because the NASA study has already established the efficiency ratio between rebounding and treadmill jogging. The tests (Balke protocol) were given between 1970 and 1981 to people who received a preventive medical examination at the Cooper Clinic.

By the end of 1985, after 100,482 person-years of follow-up (ex. if 20 people were studied for 2 years each, they would equal 40 person-years), 283 of the tested people had died. Blair and his team then calculated the number of deaths per 10,000 persons per year for each fitness level and age group. They also made calculations for groupings defined by combinations of fitness levels with other important risk factors such as smoking, blood pressure, family history, etc.

The findings of the study are age adjusted and summarized as follows. There is a strong relationship between fitness and mortality rates. The greater the fitness the greater the effect of the relationship between fitness and mortality. The mortality rate decreased as the fitness level increased. Fitness had this same protective action regardless of age. Even moderate levels of physical fitness protect against early death.

That part about even moderate levels of exercise providing protection really caught my eye.

The study assigned each participant to one of five levels of fitness. The one fifth that stayed on the treadmill the longest was assigned to the fittest or category 5. The one fifth that stayed on the least was assigned category 1, with categories 2, 3 and 4, equally divided between them.

Blair's team looked at each fitness level in combination with other risk factors for early death to see whether the fitness benefit was active in spite of the other health reducing conditions. They specifically analyzed the interaction of fitness level with blood pressure, cholesterol level, blood glucose level, cigarette smoking, body mass index and family history.

They found that for each of these 5 risk categories, improved fitness significantly reduced early mortality.

The most dramatic protection gains were achieved by moving out of category 1 into category 2 or 3. The study's most striking example was among women with high blood pressure. Just by improving to fitness category 2, a woman would improve her chances of survival by *18.28 times* better relative risk (that's 1,828%). Another one of the most striking examples appeared in Blair's study when combining fitness and fatness categories in men. But once again, the moving out of category 1 to category 2 or 3, even if one is still obese, improved the chances of survival by 300%!

The report stated that "Higher levels of physical fitness appear to delay all-cause mortality...primarily due to lowered rates of cardiovascular disease and cancer."

When an increase in fitness is combined with the rest of the Healthy Cell Concept—proper cellular health, exercise, and environment—even greater protection is achieved. Remember, the above study was done on treadmills. NASA says rebounding is as much as 68% more efficient than treadmill jogging. Therefore, moving from category 1 to category 2 or 3 of fitness levels for both men and women can be achieved by rebounding only 3–5 minutes twice a day, just as long as one of those minutes the person is performing the aerobic bounces as vigorous as they can go.

From the studies presented above it is clear that The Executive Fitness Program I presented ten years ago to all Executives who would listen has now been vindicated by scientific studies.

"What Executive Fitness Program?" I hear you asking.

I will be glad to present it to you right now in its entirety.

> ## THE REBOUND EXERCISE
> ## EXECUTIVE FITNESS PROGRAM.
> - Rebound doing the Health Bounce for 30 seconds.
> - Continue rebounding by doing the Strength Bounce for 1 minute.
> - Rebound Sprint as fast as you can by lifting your knees up in front of you and swinging your arms for 1 minute.
> - Warm down by doing the Health Bounce for 1 minute.
> - Repeat the above once in the morning once at night.
>
>   These seven minutes a day will provide you with all of the exercise you need to dramatically increase the quality and longevity of your life.

Bob Hope lived to see his one hundredth birthday. His rebounder, that he used faithfully for over fifteen years, was at the foot of his bed. I will see you on the other side of one hundred years.

It was a beautiful spring day so, rather than rebounding, I decided to jog around my neighborhood. Less than a block from my house, an empty beer can was hurled at me from a passing automobile filled with fun loving teenagers. The empty aluminum projectile missed me and probably would not have hurt much even if it hit me but it made me angry.

While still fuming at the thoughtlessness of the truant ones, I did not notice that a gate in the middle of a fence was left slightly ajar—an opportunity that was immediately apparent to the resident guard dog. I thought nothing of the barking ruckus as I ran past his yard until suddenly he was ferociously nipping at my heels. Out of sheer fright and desperation, I leaped onto the hood of the closest parked car and did not stop until I was sitting on the middle of the roof. And there I stayed until the owner of the dog and the automobile,came out to apologize and closed the gate behind his dog.

As I walked home I had an even greater appreciation for rebound exercise. I finished my exercise for the day on my rebounder as I contemplated that I did not have to subject myself to barking and biting dogs, irresponsible acts of other people, rain, sleet, snow, traffic, muggings, mud puddles, mailboxes, summer heat, etc.

Why was I jogging out there anyway? I knew better. I knew that jogging subjected the body to bone jarring trauma which eventually manifests itself in shin splints, ankle problems, knee problems and lower back problems. Rebounding eliminates most of the trauma while providing an aerobic experience.

There I was, finishing my exercise in the comforts and conveniences of my own air conditioned family room, in front of my television, surrounded by my family and engaged in enjoyable conversation. When I got off the rebounder to get a drink of water, my daughter mounted the unit and rebounded. Eventually, she got off and my wife took advantage of the vacant mat. She relinquished the rebounder when a football game came on the television because she knew I enjoyed playing along with our football team. They ran up and down the field, and I kept up with them by rebounding.

What a way to get your one-a-day multiple exercise program! Rebounding is fun, easy, convenient, economical and safe. It builds balance coordination, rhythm and timing while building muscle bulk and strength. Take this form of exercise, slide it in front of a television and you will understand why more and more people are turning on to rebound exercise.

Rebound exercise equipment comes in different shapes and sizes

People involved with consistent, habitual exercise programs find when they cannot exercise for any reason it just about drives them crazy! Athletes who are injured to the point of being bedridden find this condition is intolerable.

It is possible those who have chosen rebound exercise as their exercise mode find that not being able to rebound is simply unacceptable. I know, I have been in those situations. I seldom travel without bringing a rebounder with me so I can open it up in the hotel room. I have even opened a rebounder to exercise in an airborne Boeing 747 between Hong Kong and the United States. I thought I was really in trouble when the copilot came back to the cabin area where I was rebounding, until he asked if he could rebound for a few minutes too. There have been too many times that I turned hotel beds into oversize rebounders.

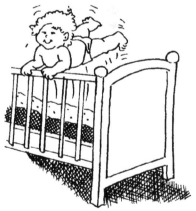

Have you noticed children jump up and down on anything and everything including brothers and sisters? Jumping appears to be a very natural phenomenon and quite possibly vitally important as a

Jumping seems to be a very natural movement, children and even adults will often jump on any available springy surface.

child begins to develop muscle control and basic balance techniques. Beds, tree branches, fast moving elevators, pogo sticks, springboards and diving boards all provide some degree of rebound exercise. But because these devices are not designed for the specific purpose of providing rebound exercise, they can not be relied upon for a satisfactory rebound exercise program.

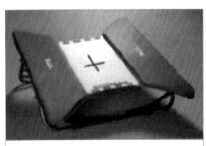

Mini-trampolines are small angled trampolines. Gymnasts take a running start and jump onto the mat catapulting themselves into the air in order to better perform gymnastic feats.

The mini-trampoline, a gymnastic device, cannot be used as a source of rebound exercise. That is because the bed of the mini-trampoline is set at a diagonal so, the gymnast can run and bounce once and be catapulted into the air to perform gymnastics. The gymnast lands on a crash pad or some other gymnastic device. Those people who are unfamiliar with gymnastics many times confuse a mini-trampoline with the rebounder. They call a rebounder a mini-trampoline, and vice versa.

It is possible to use a trampoline as a rebound device. NASA did it as they studied the difference between rebound exercise and treadmill jogging. Gymnasts, divers and snow skiers have used the trampoline for years to keep in shape. In reality, the trampoline is a platform for tricks to be used by acrobats, gymnasts and circus performers for the purpose of learning or performing tricks. One of the benefits of trampolining is rebound exercise.

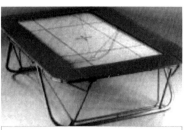

Trampolines can be fun to jump on and can be great for gymnastics. They are not ideal exercise for everyone, however.

In the early 1980s, there were only five companies who were manufacturing rebound exercise equipment. By 1983, we were able to identify over 100 different United States manufacturers producing exercise equipment with the rebound exercise concept in mind. It was crazy! Some were square made of angle iron with four legs, 48 weak springs and a canvas mat. Others had six sides and six legs. Then there were the oval and rectangular frames. One was called the grasshopper. It was 54 inches in diameter, painted green, had a plastic mat 60 springs and eight legs. Surprisingly it had a good bounce. But it was too big and clumsy to fit inside a family room.

Ah, those were the good old days of experimentation and investigation. One rebound device was simply a truck tire inner tube supporting fish netting. If you wanted to change the bounce you simply added more air to the truck tire. There were long springs, short springs, weak springs, strong springs and even shock cords used to support the various mats, which were made out of canvas, plastic, nylon, fishnets and eventually Permatron™.

Now, there is a fabric! It is usually black or blue, impervious to the weather, extremely strong and it does not stretch! The use of Permatron™ was a revolutionary breakthrough in the rebound exercise industry because now the mats don't stretch out of shape. The entire bounce comes from the springs, where the bounce should come from. Eventually by guess, by golly and by experimentation, we determined the best configuration was a round frame. That is probably because a circle is the strongest structure in a single plane. The circular shape allows all of the springs to support the mat equally.

For a young industry, everything seemed to be going the way it should. The National Institute of Reboundology and Health was selling about 25,000 books a month to thousands of distributors and hundreds of manufacturers. Then I received four disturbing phone calls all in one week. Each from a different manufacturer; each claiming to have secured the contract to supply rebounders to the same large chain of department stores. It was obvious not all of these reports could be right.

What really happened was that major chain of department stores was playing the four manufacturers against each other to see which one would provide the best rebounder at the best possible price. The manufacturers did not realize they were in competition with each other. Eventually all four manufacturers lost because of the invasion of third-world manufacturers.

The industry was growing so fast it caught the attention of the nation's mass merchandisers, department stores and many sporting goods stores. This would have been good for the industry except it also caught the attention of foreign merchant spies from third-world countries, who informed the mass merchandisers that they could produce round "springy thingys" cheaper than could be produced in the United States. Soon, cheap rebounder knockoffs were being advertised in the newspapers for $49.95 as a lost leader or come on. The knockoffs were made of the cheapest material, but the buyers of the mass merchandisers did not know any better, nor did they care and apparently, neither did the customers.

> "I have been using the cheap Wal-Mart trampoline, not knowing that so much research and improved rebounders were available. I recently house-sat for a friend for a month and used her reboundair. The difference sold me!"
>
> Sandra Smith, Wendell, MA

Unfortunately, the U. S. manufacturers of the quality rebound exercise equipment could not compete with the foreign cheap junk and the advertising campaign of the mass marketers so, they simply went out of business. For a decade, from 1985–1995 the rebound exercise industry was in the toilet. This was a frustrating time for us because we watched people buy the cheap rebounders expecting to receive rebound benefits and thirty to forty-five days later, the knockoffs were broken.

However, you cannot keep a good idea hidden from the public forever. There were enough people who had purchased their rebounders before 1985 who knew the difference between quality merchandise and schlock. They demanded quality and were willing to pay for it. Those die-hard manufacturers who decided to weather the storm were forced to tighten up their belts produce quality rebounders or get out of the business. So, although it was painful it was a good growing up and maturing experience for the survivors and the rebound exercise industry. You, the consumer, win.

Chapter Fifteen

Revolution, Evolution
and Innovation

The first major innovative breakthrough in the design of rebound exercise equipment came in 1985. I was a paid consultant to the Hong Kong Government to help them solve their exercise problems for 7,000 firemen and 28,000 policemen. Rebound exercise was presented as a solution to their problem at the highest level.

Hilton Cheon Ling, Chairman of the Hong Kong Government was presented the concept of rebound exercise in May of 1985. He accepted the concept but rejected the equipment. It was too bulky. He demanded that engineers on the payroll of the Hong Kong government work with me to design a folding rebounder that could be used by the Hong Kong police and fire departments.

I presented to them 38 inch rebounders with six legs solidly welded to the frame. It was state of the art at the time but its size could not be reduced. It took up too much room when it wasn't being used. That was unacceptable to the Hong Kong Government because space was such a premium in an overcrowded population.

I met with the engineers the next morning and after watching the engineers for a couple of hours, one turned the rebounder upside down. He began to enthusiastically explain his idea to the other two in Chinese. He told them he would create two off centered hinges, so the rebounder had to be turned upside down in order for it to be folded. The off centered hinges made it so the springs holding the mat in place would create tension on the frame in its unfolded position. This would prevent the frame from folding up accidentally while in use.

One of the engineers winked at me, grabbed a hacksaw and began

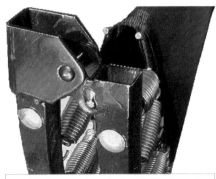

cutting the rebounder in half. Another grabbed some scrap metal and the third fired up the welder. In less then half an hour, they presented to me a rebounder that actually folded up. But that exposed an even greater problem. The legs, solidly welded to the frame, would not allow the rebounder to fold. They must come off. And so they did. 15 minutes later, the rebounder had no legs. But before the day was over six new legs were screwed on to six welded studs.

This first version of a half-fold rebounder hinge was a dramatic improvement in convenience, but still left much to be expected with regards to safety.

And in their own special way the engineers began to congratulate each other on a job well done.

The next morning we agreed screw on legs were not acceptable for two reasons. One, anything that can be screwed on can be screwed up. Two, there is the chance that if six legs are loose and you need to screw the legs on you will only be able to find five. A six legged rebounder, with only five legs is useless. "Back to the drawing board."

This time, the engineers outdid themselves. With some milling, drilling and welding they finally produced a half-fold rebounder with legs that were held in place by springs on the inside of the legs, so that the legs were permanently attached. This reduced the possibility of losing them. They simply snapped into position over the welded studs.

Before presenting the half-fold rebounder with spring-loaded folding legs to Hilton Cheon Ling, the

Rachel Kranz, said in an e-mail to our team:

"It's wonderful!!! I LOVE it!!! I'm so pleased to have this great way of exercising right in my own home, and I'm REALLY glad I have the easy-to-use half-fold. Thank you SO MUCH for your patience and help with the whole process of getting started; you have my sincere gratitude both for your helpfulness and for the rebounder itself. I know I'll get a lot of use out of it, and my health, spirits, and fitness levels will all benefit. THANKS again for service and kindness above and beyond the call of duty.

Gratefully,
Rachel"

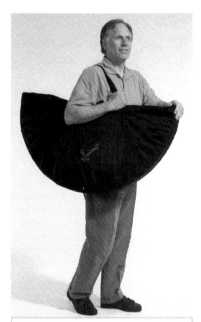

The custom crafted carrying case of the Half-Fold ReboundAIR makes for convenient storage or travel.

next morning they designed and sewed a carrying case to demonstrate how easy it would be to carry and store. The Chairman of the Hong Kong government was very pleased with his engineers. Quite frankly, I was amazed because I did not think it could be done.

Also, the concept of six spring-loaded legs attached to the frame by one inch studs was so appealing we decided to use this revolution on our standard non folding rebounder. Instead of needing a box that was 40 inches by 40 inches by 8inches, we could now ship them in a box 40 X 20 X 4. It was a major breakthrough in shipping and storing rebounders.

When my time in Hong Kong came to a close, I was presented a half-fold rebounder and was given permission to market it anyplace in the world except Hong Kong. I was unable to patent the idea but the concept has caught on. Today at least five companies manufacture a half-fold rebounder and some of them even produce non-folding rebounders with springs in the legs.

The Evolution of the Safety Hinge used Exclusively on the Half-Fold ReboundAIR

Although we sold thousands of Half-Fold rebounders the first few years, I could see there were some problems. I did not like that you had to pull the frame cover off the hinges before folding the rebounder or the hinge would tear a hole right through the frame cover. If you unfolded the unit on a shag carpet the hinge would grab the shag carpet making it impossible to lift the rebounder without ruining the carpet. If the frame cover slipped over the hinge while it was

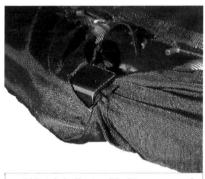

Old style bulky jaw-like hinges can grab anything in their path from spring covers, to carpets or even little fingers.

unfolding, the rebounder would grab the frame cover. Also, it looked dangerous. I have never heard of anybody getting their fingers caught in the hinge and it is a good thing because it could cause some real damage.

After receiving numerous calls from people requesting a new frame cover because they didn't pull it away from the hinges, I decided something had to be done. I bought a few pieces of balsa wood and began to carve an acceptable hinge, one that would be friendly to the frame cover and any fingers that accidentally got in the way.

Not being a mechanical engineer myself, I took the new wooden hinge and the folding rebounder to the Department of Mechanical Engineering at Brigham Young University. It was a good project for them and soon they had produced an aluminum hinge. It had merit.

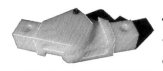

Nylon model of the safety hinge designed by Al Carter.

I took the hinge with me to my factory. The engineers actually got excited about it and within a week had produced a nylon hinge that did not have to be welded. They said it could be inserted into the square steel tube frame and held snugly in place by the already existing clevis pins which connect the springs to the frame. This way if there was any problem with the hinge it could be easily replaced. Then we tested it. We folded the frame and I put my finger right on top of the hinge and unfolded the unit. The unfolding hinge pushed my finger away! We put the frame cover on the frame and folded the unit and it did not hurt the frame cover at all!

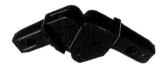

Safety hinges push objects away as they close so that carpets, spring covers and fingers are safe.

The next step was to produce the hinge. We found a casting factory that agreed to produce them for a price. I paid the money and bought the cast. So, now I own the casts for the hinge. The casts are at the foundry, but the only folding rebounders which have the Safety Hinge are the ones with the ReboundAIR logo on them.

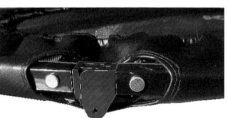

The safety hinge bolts securely into the frame.

The year 1986 found me brainstorming all over the United States and Canada with my half-fold rebounder that I was able to take with me as airplane carry-on luggage. If nothing else it was is an excellent conversation piece at the airports.

It was about that time I began to question whether a rebounder could be folded again to make it even more compact without destroying its integrity. The idea was daunting. Where some people would fold paper airplanes, I caught myself making folding rebounders out of paper and trying to fold them again.

I believe I can tell you all of the ways the rebounder can not be folded in fourths because I probably tried them all. My garage was filled with bits and pieces of failed quarter-fold rebounders.

It was not until I went back to the Engineering Department of Brigham Young University, Provo, Utah, and explained my plight that I finally got the results I was looking

"Dear Mr. Carter,

I recently purchased one of your quarter-folding [Ultimate Rebound] mini trampolines and I've been wanting to thank you ever since. My only excuse for not doing so before is that I spend all my spare time on it.

...You should have seen the grin on my face. And the way my body felt!

...It's literally the best purchase I've made for myself in the past 15 years, definitely the one I feel the happiest about.

for. Six months after I presented the problem to them they had the solution in CAD drawing form. Now, all I had to do was find a manufacturer someplace in the world that would be willing to take a chance on an idea whose time had come. Luckily we did.

That composite quarter-fold Ultimate Rebound exerciser is now patented and in full production. Our most innovative and convenient quarter-fold design is a revolutionary breakthrough in rebounding design. Unlike any other rebounder on the market, it is constructed with the latest in composite polymer material used in aircraft and high performance automobile engines. The composite polymer frame is stronger yet lighter than metal frames. The legs unlock and fold stowing

Now the best built most innovative rebounder on the planet can be folded and transported for the busy professional or the rebound enthusiast alike.

perfectly into the frame. The frame folds twice to fit inside the custom carrying case, then slides snugly onto the durable luggage dolly for ultimate convenience and portability. Health club quality at an in home price. It's excellent for demonstrations, traveling, physical therapists or those who want the most state-of-the-art rebounding equipment. Aggressively tested by a 300 pound user, this Ultimate Rebound comes with a lifetime warranty for users up to 400 pounds.

Other Rebound Equipment

The question is often asked, "What other equipment do you need besides a quality rebounder to participate in a complete rebound exercise program?" The answer is simple. "Nothing."

You do not need special shoes, socks, special rebound tights, halter tops or T-shirts. In fact, anything else you want to bring to your rebound area is up to you and your particular circumstances.

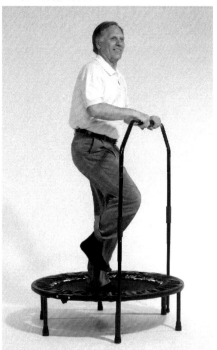

If you do not trust your balance while rebounding you may enjoy rebounding with some extra support. My first recommendation is a wall. Slide the rebounder up next to a wall, so you can put one or both hands on the wall to provide the support you need while you rebound. Then you can enjoy excellent exercise and gradually wean yourself away from the wall. Because rebound exercise stimulates the vestibular system, under normal circumstances you can expect it to improve your balance, so that you will no longer need to touch the wall for support.

If you feel the need for more stability than the wall can offer, you may want to use a stabilizing bar that attaches to two of the legs of the rebounder. These stabilizing bars provide support no matter what level of rebound exercise you do.

A stability bar can give you confidence while rebounding as a beginner or even a more advanced bouncer.

Although weights are not necessary to develop the upper body while rebounding, they do enhance the process. We will give some suggestions as to how to use weights when we talk about Aerobic Resistive Rebounding. We recommend two different types of weights. Our one pound or three pound one size fits all glove weights fit on to the back of the hands with Velcro around the wrists. These give you complete use of your hands to hold on to a balance bar, the back of a chair or even other handheld weights. They also prevent dumbbell-to-chin collisions.

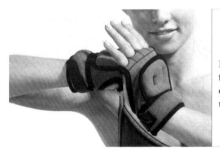

Rebounding with weights is called Aerobic Resistive Rebounding. The weights enhance the workout by making it more intense. They especially help to intensify the workout for the upper body.

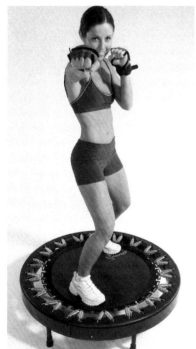

These convenient hand weights will not slip out of your hands during a workout. They make shadow boxing an even better workout.

One, two and three pound hand-held weights are also popular around rebounders. However, care should be taken as you rebound with steel weights. Make sure you do not hit yourself, somebody close by or lose control and let them fly.

For those of you who are interested in improving your vision, the Enhance your Vision with Rebound Exercise kit is available. Do not forget that your eyes are part of your body also and have the ability of becoming stronger cell by cell with the cellular exercise available by rebounding.

If you are home schooling your preschoolers, there is no better tool available than the Rebound Education Kit and a good rebounder. Systematically learn the symbols of civilization (colors, numbers, shapes and the alphabet), while enhancing balance, coordination, rhythm, timing, dexterity and kinesthetic awareness. These are prerequisite skills one has to have before the end of the first grade or one is considered a delayed learner. Rebounding is a great way to get the entire body involved in the learning process.

If you do not like to exercise alone, then may we suggest a rebound exercise workout video or DVD. Turn it on and enjoy an organized strategically controlled exercise program. Then there are people who like to go at their own speed so, they bounce at their own pace to their favorite music. All that is needed is the right rhythm and the right time when you are in the right exercise mood.

Exercise experts all over the world are beginning to realize the validity, simplicity and convenience of rebound exercise. Many clubs and spas are beginning to offer rebound exercise classes.

The American Institute of Reboundology Inc. periodically offers Reboundology Seminars, making it possible for those serious about rebounding to become Certified Reboundologists™. Now this opportunity is being made available through a newly released distance learning DVD. There are now thousands of Certified Reboundologists™ spreading the good news of cellular exercise, and you can be one of them. For information about the Certification Seminar or any other ReboundAIR products visit www. ReboundAIR.com or call 1(888)464-JUMP (5867).

Chapter Sixteen

Rebound Moves and Activities

Today, most rebounders are able to be folded either at the legs or at the legs and the frame. So, before mounting any rebounder always check to make sure all legs are secured in their proper place. When you are setting up the legs, it is easy to secure five out of six legs and to leave the leg farthest from you unsecure.

When Certified Reboundologists call in to AIR, Inc. to ask technical and health questions, it is important that we are able to communicate and understand the various moves on the rebounder. This is why we have classified the moves as the strength, aerobic and health bounces. Now, we realize the lymphatic system becomes very active in any rebound exercise, making all of the bounces healthy. Cellular strength is increased with virtually any rebounding building strength with each bounce. These classifications of the exercises are helpful for communication purposes, and have been beneficial in the rebound industry.

The Health Bounce

If you are unsure of your balance, make sure the rebounder is next to a wall or has a stabilizing bar properly attached. For balance, place your hands on the wall or grasp the balance bar. Step up onto the mat of the rebounder. Position yourself in the center of the mat with your feet about six inches apart. Begin bouncing on your toes by bending your knees and straightening them or shrugging your shoulders. Doing the health bounce

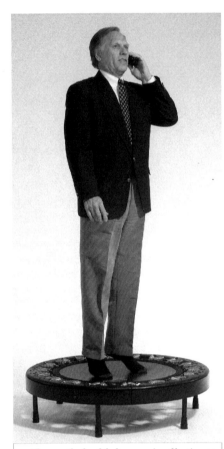

The gentle health bounce is effective at increasing lymphatic circulation as well as giving you a needed energy boost in the middle of the day. This is a move which is useful for beginner through advanced bouncers.

does not require your feet to leave the mat. Continue this activity for three to five minutes or as long as it is comfortable. There it is. That is the health bounce. That's all there is to it!

Now, if you step off from the rebounder, notice that you are tingling all over. That tingling is in part because the lymphatic system has been turned on. The millions of one-way valves have been activated and metabolic garbage has been sucked out from around the tissue spaces, providing a healthier environment for all of the cells of your body. That is why it is called the health bounce.

The up and down activity of the simple health bounce challenges the function of the vestibular system, the neurotransmitters in the brainstem and the antigravity muscles. You are beginning to develop a keener sense of balance.

As you oscillate on the rebounder your eyes have to constantly focus on various objects in the room challenging the minute visual muscles. You are beginning to improve your vision.

Although very simple, the health bounce will probably be used more than all of the other bounces combined because it will be the bounce you will use for your warm up and your cool down for every rebound exercise workout.

Aerobic Bounces

All of the aerobic bounces are designed to challenge the oxygen delivery systems, the cardiopulmonary and vascular systems, including the heart, lungs, arteries and veins.

Rebound Walk

In the center of the rebounder after you have warmed up with the health bounce, begin walking in place lifting your knees up in front of you one at a time, while leaning back slightly. This is an exercise you can do for several minutes.

Rebound Jog

In the center of the rebounder after you have warmed up with the health bounce or the rebound walk, begin jogging in place by lifting your knees higher in front of you one at a time, while leaning back slightly. As your left knee comes up, swing your right arm forward in front of you. As your right knee comes up, swing your left arm forward. Concentrate on breathing deeply.

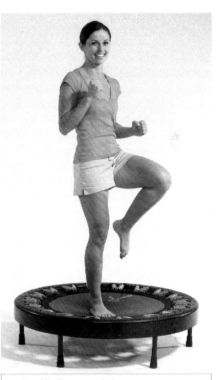

The largest muscles of your body, those in your arms, abdomen and legs are using up the available oxygen in your bloodstream replacing it with carbon dioxide. This creates an oxygen debt. The oxygen is replaced in the process when your heartbeat increases in strength and speed. This increases bloodflow to the part of the body with oxygen debt.

Aerobic bounces help to create oxygen debt in your body by using some of the largest muscles in the body. This rebound jog is a bounce which can be adapted for anyone from beginners to advanced.

Continue the rebound jog for a few minutes or as long as it is comfortable. Always finish your rebounding with the health bounce.

Rebound Run

The rebound run can be performed in two body positions. The first one is just like the rebound jog only faster. The second one, instead of leaning backward, you lean forward and kick your legs out behind you. Swing your right arm forward as you kick your left leg back and vice versa. Continue to concentrate on breathing deeply.

The rebound run is a more strenuous move, so, you will probably be able to do it for a shorter duration than the rebound jog. Be sure to cool down with the health bounce to minimize the buildup of lactic acid in the muscles. It is the buildup of lactic acid that makes the muscles sore the next morning.

Rebound Sprint

This is the kicker. It is performed just like the rebound jog, only as fast as you can go. You will usually sandwich it in between the rebound run or the rebound jog. You will probably Rebound Sprint for only about 50–250 steps. The Rebound Sprint will cause you to use all of your lung capacity. Be sure to concentrate on breathing deeply.

Rebound Cross Crawl

While doing the rebound jog, bring your right elbow down to touch your left knee as it comes up, then bring your left elbow down to touch your right knee. Besides being a good exercise this is an excellent activity for children with poor motor skills or learning disabilities.

Rebound High Kick Forward

This one is fun. Lean backwards to maintain your balance, kick your left leg straight out in front of you as high as you can kick. Then on the next bounce, kick your right leg straight out. Swing your arms in rhythm with the kicks to keep your balance.

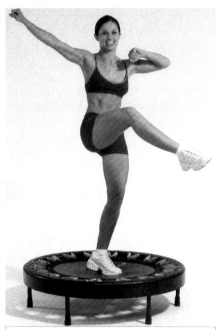

As you kick your legs out in front of you, try pointing your toes up. Notice the effect it has on the calves of your legs. Next try pointing your toes straight out. Then change by pointing your toes up sometimes and pointing them out at other times.

Rebound High Kick Backward

Now try the high step backward by leaning forward and kicking your

The high kick is an intense aerobic bounce that can help you to firm up and feel great. It is an intermediate to advanced move.

legs out behind you. You may have to swing your arms on this one just to maintain your balance.

Rebound High Kick Sideways

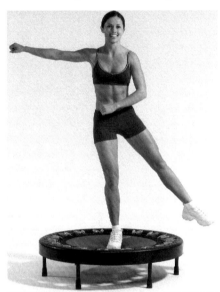

This aerobic bounce helps you to intensify the workout for your abs and obliques. It is a moderate to advanced move.

Try kicking your legs out to the side one at a time. You will have to lean to the opposite direction from the kick to maintain your balance. This will create a rocking motion in the upper body.

As soon as you feel you have mastered the high kicks, try putting them all together; the front kicks, the back kicks and the side-kicks, each time landing in the center of the rebounder. You might even notice your balance and your vision improving while carrying on these activities. Besides being in better shape, your improvement in balance and vision will benefit you all the way up to your next rebounding session.

The Strength Bounces

By definition, a strength bounce is when both feet leave the mat at the same time. The strength bounce requires you to use the rebounder like a trampoline without the tricks.

A visit to your local health club will expose you to the old-fashioned way of developing strength. It is slow, cumbersome and dangerous. The strength bounces are classified as such because we have found that G loading the body with the rebound exercise will strengthen every cell in the body and thus the entire body benefits. Sir Isaac Newton discovered the formula for the pull of gravity and its relationship to acceleration to a free falling body. The formula is 32 feet per second per second. When you bounce and your feet leave the mat, after you pass the apex of the bounce, you become a free falling body in the earth's gravitational pull for a fraction of a second. So, the higher you jump, the greater will be the speed when you land on the rebounder again, increasing gravity or creating a greater G-Force. All of the cells of the body dutifully do what they are supposed to do, which is simply to adjust to the increased gravity and greater stimulation by becoming stronger. Because of this phenomenon, a high strength bounce has a much different affect on the body than a low strength bounce.

Rebound Shuffle Bounce

After warming up with the health bounce, jump higher. The springs will push you into the air so both feet leave the mat. Land with one foot forward and one foot back. On the next bounce change foot positions. The muscles used to push the toes into the mat are the calf muscles. Because of this, many people find their calf muscles become tired long before they want to stop rebounding. The shuffle bounce allows you to land on the heel of one foot and your toes of the other, so you do not overtax your calf muscles before you've completed your rebounding. You will find you will be able to rebound much longer by incorporating the shuffle bounce into your routine.

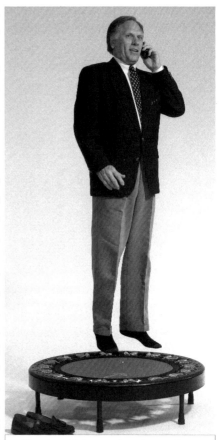

The strength bounce is a vigorous bounce which stimulates lymphatic circulation while producing a high cell-strengthening G-Force at the bottom of the bounce.

Low Strength Bounce

The low strength bounce is done the same way as the health bounce, but like all strength bounces, you bounce high enough so your feet leave the mat. The low strength bounce is used primarily to change your body positions on the rebounder. Now you are able to turn every time you bounce.

Try turning to the right just a little bit each time you bounce, so you are eventually facing another wall. Now, each time you bounce, turn to the left until several bounces later you are back where you started. Continue bouncing to the left until you have turned all the way around. You will find this turning technique can be used to enhance your balance and make your workout more fun.

While you are using the turning method, try turning 90 degrees to the right with a single bounce. When you accomplish that, do it again. Do it two more times and you are back where you started.

This time turn 90 degrees to the left then do it three more times.

Now turn to the right by 90 degrees, then to the left by 90 degrees. Then throw in the 90 degree turns in random order.

As soon as you are comfortable with the 90 degree turns begin planning for your 180 degree turns. Jump higher; you may need a little more altitude. Jump and turn at the same time, so you land facing the opposite direction. Duplicate that move several times until it feels comfortable. Then jump and turn the other direction by 180 degrees.

Each time you turn by 90 degrees or 180 degrees it requires your eyes to focus on another part of the room. This sends a report back to your brain telling it exactly where you are. This reorientation each time you bounce stimulates and exercises the eyes.

The turning bounces also stimulate the vestibular system, which in turn, dramatically improves your balance and coordination. You will find this added balance is not only available to you while you are rebounding but is there to enhance all other physical activities afterward.

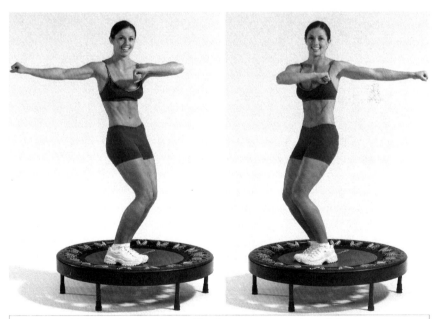

This fun moderate to intermediate bounce can give a dance feel to your workout. It also intensifies the workout for your obliques and abs.

The Slalom Bounce

Skiers and wannabe skiers, hold on to your goggles, your ski poles and your gloves. This next exercise is for all who enjoy the slopes.

Start with a low strength bounce and landing with both feet left of the center of the mat with the toes pointed towards the centerline. The next landing would be on the right of the center of the mat of the rebounder with the toes pointed towards the centerline. Your body should be in a crouched position facing forward with your hands holding imaginary ski poles at shoulder level out in front and slightly to the side. Your legs and feet bounce rapidly from side to side. All of the activity should be below the waist with your upper body hardly moving at all. The balance, coordination and physical fitness developed by doing the slalom bounce is phenomenal! It is the exercise we need during the summer to prepare for the slopes in the winter.

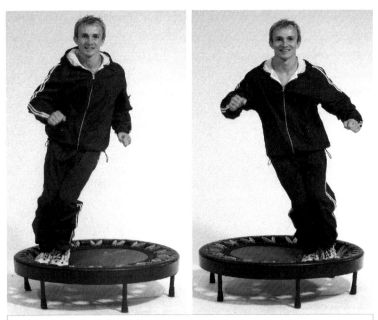

This energetic addition to the workout helps you to prepare for
the slopes. It is an advanced addition to your workout.

The Twist Bounce

The twist bounce is done by landing with the lower body turned one direction and the upper body turned facing the opposite direction. The directions are reversed with the next bounce.

Most back pain occurs in the lower part of the back about the fifth lumbar vertabra. The twist bounce strengthens this area of the back reducing the potential of lower back pain.

The High Strength Bounce

There's no better way to G load the entire body all at once than with the high strength bounce. The primary purpose for the high strength bounce is to strengthen every cell in the body. This is accomplished by jumping as high as you can, landing in the center of the rebounder to jump again.

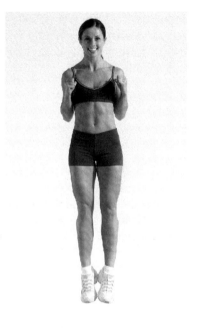

To get the greatest amount of altitude with each bounce you need to shove your toes into the mat while straightening your knees and your hips and thrusting your arms rapidly into the air.

According to the United States Air Force, the normal healthy body is able to withstand 10Gs when the body is in a vertical position. So, the maximum of 3.24Gs developed by rebounding as high as you can go is well with in the safe parameters for a healthy human body. If you feel your body is not in the best physical condition, we suggest you do not try to bounce as high as you can. Bounce more gently, to keep the G-Force on your body under 3Gs. Just to help you estimate, if you bounced so your feet are four to six inches off the mat you would be creating approximately a G-Force of 2Gs.

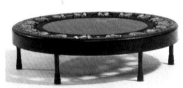

The high strength bounce helps you to optimize the stacking of G-force while rebounding. When doing the high strength bounce your body may experience as much as 3.5 times the normal force of gravity.

Rebound Dancing

We have presented to you many various bounces you can do on the rebounder and we have explained some of the benefits of each bounce. You will notice however, we have said very little about upper body movements. If you feel we have slighted that part of your physical anatomy, now is our time to rectify that.

Go get a CD of your favorite be-bop, '60s, '70s and '80s dance tunes, your favorite jazz music or a good classical CD. Insert it into your player, turn the volume up slightly, mount your rebounder and be prepared to envelop yourself totally and completely into a fantastic new way of toning and tightening your body. With rebound dancing let your imagination soar using all of the moves we have presented to you, including the shuffling, jogging or running, high kicks and turning bounces. Create your own choreographic moves and create a better you. The sky is the limit—literally—because there will be times you will be reaching for the sky. How about reaching for your toe in the middle of a high step? Try a turn, high step, turn. You may feel clumsy at first, but as you continue to practice the various moves and bounces and continue to exercise to different music you will be ecstatic with the results.

Eyes Closed

Why would anybody want to bounce on a rebounder with his or her eyes closed? The answer to that question is anybody who wants to improve his or her sense of balance. Scientists agree we not only use our eyes to see our environment, but they are also major balancing mechanisms. We view vertical lines, horizontal lines and diagonal lines and adjust our body positions, according to our viewed perceptions. At least 80% of everything we learn about our environment comes to us through our eyes, including our posture.

However, if we close our eyes, then we have to rely upon our other balancing mechanisms in order to maintain our upright position. The bouncing motion stimulates the nerves of the foot pads on the bottom of your feet to determine whether the weight is distributed on your toes, heels, right or left foot. This challenges the antigravity muscles at every bounce and forces the vestibular system to work faster and more accurately. I believe I could ask the question, "Who needs better balance?" And virtually everyone would admit that a keener sense of balance would be very beneficial.

There are several techniques you can use to develop better balance on a rebounder. First, simply begin your rebound routine and close your eyes. Open them immediately if you feel you are off balance. Or, use the stabilizing bar and close your eyes while rebounding and take your hands off the balance bar. Immediately grasp the bar if you feel off balance. An easy third way to do this is to put the rebounder next to a wall and touch the wall with your hands. Close your eyes and move your hand away from the wall. If you begin to loose your balance, touch the wall and open your eyes. Continue the practice of closing your eyes while you rebounding until you can rebound your entire routine without the use of your eyes.

As part of his preparation for wrestling competition, I would have Darren rebound with his eyes closed. I even had him wear a hooded sweatshirt backwards with the hood up over his head and tied behind his neck. The results, were remarkable. On the wrestling mat he had such a catlike sense of balance his opponents could not take him down. I am sure rebounding with his eyes closed was part of the reason he became Washington State's Wrestling Champion five times and National Wrestling Champion twice.

Sitting Bounce

The sitting bounce is probably the most famous bounce, because it has been featured on the front cover of *The Miracles of Rebound Exercise*. Still, it is probably the least understood of all of the bounces. Many different people in various health and physical conditions use it for all sorts of reasons. From children watching television all the way to serious abdominal crunches by the best athletes.

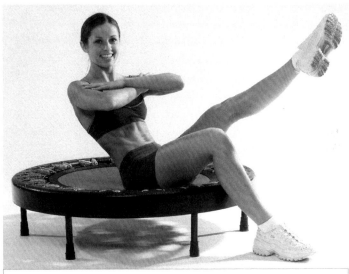

This sitting bounce is a beginning to moderate ab exercise.

Sit down as close to the center of the rebounder as you can with your feet comfortably positioned on the floor in front of you. Begin your bouncing motion by shrugging your shoulders and moving your arms up and down rhythmically. Or, create the bounce by holding onto the frame and pushing down on it. Your body will move upward as you rhythmically push on the frame. Some people prefer to put their hands on the mat beside them and push off from the mat to create the bounce. Still others do not have the ability to create a bounce by themselves. In these cases, the bounce can be created by a person health bouncing on the mat behind the person sitting.

There are several positions which can be used by those who are interested in developing stronger abdominal muscles. After creating a rhythmic bounce, lean back slightly and hold your knees with your hands while continuously shrugging your shoulders. You will continue to bounce. This position will challenge the abdominal and back muscles.

As you continue to bounce, release the hold on your knees and lean back a little farther. Put your hands on your abdominal muscles and feel the work they do each time you bounce.

Lift one foot up from the floor and continue to bounce. This will create the next level of abdominal exercises. Then replace that foot on the floor and lift your other leg up and continue to bounce.

V-Sit

Finally, while bouncing, lift both legs in the air so you are bouncing in a "V" position. This takes a little balance and coordination, but you'll get it. Your back and abdominal muscles will be enhanced greatly as you include this aspect of rebounding into your regular rebound exercise routine.

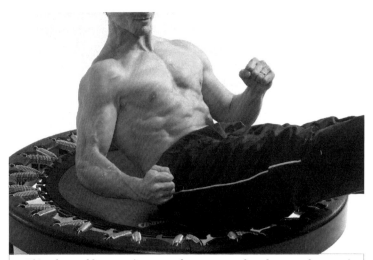

This advanced bounce gives your abs a great workout because they are the angle between your legs and upper body and they must hold the weight of your body (compounded by gravity) in place at the bottom of each bounce.

Other Applications for the Sitting Bounce

Most people who use the sitting bounces are healthy, happy and simply convinced the sitting bounces are excellent additions to the other rebound moves. Some people with injuries or disabilities also find the sitting bounce an ideal exercise for them.

The sitting bounces are excellent for those who are recovering from broken or sprained feet, ankles or legs who do not want to wait for the healing process before carrying on a regular exercise program.

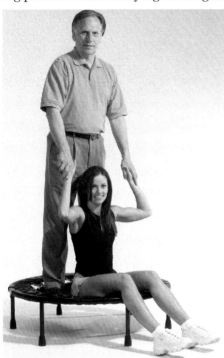

Rebound therapy provides useful lymph stimulation and exercise for paraplegics and quadriplegics who are unable to rebound alone. John provides a gentle bounce for Kara as she sits on the rebounder.

People who have chronic lower back problems also use the sitting bounces. We recommend sitting on the rebounder with your feet on the ground and bouncing gently. When you feel confident and your back is strong enough, you can lift one leg off the ground and eventually both. These exercises have a tendency to straighten out the back because gentle rebounding can strengthen the supporting muscles of the lower back. This sitting health bounce assists in the healing process.

Paraplegics, those who have no control of their lower extremities, find the sitting bounce is an ideal exercise for them. A vigorous sitting bounce helps them to get an aerobic workout, something that is often not available to them. Quadriplegics enjoy the sitting bounce also, but they need the assistance of somebody standing behind them creating a bounce and holding their upper body vertical on the rebounder so they do not tip over while rebounding.

Others who benefit from the sitting bounce are the elderly, the physically handicapped, those who have poor balance, those who are recovering from serious accidents or surgery and those who are suffering from other debilitating conditions.

Almost any athlete competing in virtually any sport can benefit from a few minutes of the sitting bounces in the various positions and intensities. If you are anywhere from a quadriplegic to a world-class athlete, you too can benefit dramatically from the sitting bounces and rebound exercise.

Chapter Seventeen

Suggested Rebound Exercise Programs

No two people are the same. Each body requires different environmental stimulation at various times in its life. The following chart is designed to take a person who has never been involved with any exercise program and help them achieve a sustainable rebound exercise activity. This is only an example of an exercise chart. If it is too simple then you 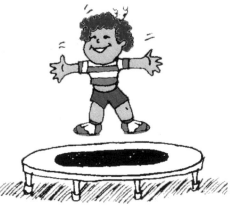 can modify it to suit your individual needs. What ever you create, it is important you stick with it.

"How soon can a child start rebounding?"

They should begin before they are born. Because rebound exercise is a cellular exercise, jumping on a rebounder will stimulate every cell in the body, including the placenta and all of the cells of the unborn child. The vestibular system and the striated muscles of the just born rebound baby will exhibit the greatest amount of his/her improvement. My grandson, Braun, walked at seven months because his mother rebounded through-

SUGGESTED BEGINNING REBOUND EXERCISE PROGRAM

	6AM 1/2 hr before breakfast	11:30AM (1/2 hr before lunch)	7:00PM (3 hr before bed)	Totals
1st week	1 min. health 1 min. aerobic	1 min. health 2 min. aerobic	1 min. health 2 min. aerobic	
5 days/wk.	2 min. total	3 min. total	3 min. total	8 min./day 40 min./wk.
2nd week	2 min. strength 2 min. health	1 min. health 3 min. aerobic	1 min. health 3 min. strength	
5 days/wk.	4 min. total	4 min. total	4 min. total	12 min./day 60 min./wk.
3rd week	1 min. health 2 min. aerobic 2 min. strength 1 min. health	1 min. health 3 min. aerobic 1 min. health	1 min. health 4 min. strength 1 min. health	
5 days/wk.	6 min. total	5 min. total	6 min. total	17 min./day 85 min./wk.
4th week	2 min. health 3 min. aerobic 3 min. strength 1 min. health	2 min. health 4 min. aerobic 1 min. health	2 min. health 4 min. strength 4 min. aerobic 1 min. health	
5 days/wk.	9 min. total	7 min. total	11 min. total	27 min./day 135 min./wk.
5th week	2 min. health 5 min. aerobic 4 min. strength 1 min. health	2 min. health 4 min. aerobic 3 min. strength 1 min. health	2 min. health 5 min. aerobic 4 min. strength 1 min. health	
5 days/wk.	12 min. total	10 min. total	12 min. total	34 min./day 170 min./wk.

out her entire pregnancy including even the day of his birth. After he was born, his mother would wrap him gently and hold him as she mounted the rebounder and gently health-bounced him to sleep. It is interesting that even if a mother does not have the rebounder she usually will rebound the baby by jostling him/her up and down in effort to get him/her to take a nap. The health bounce on the rebounder is much easier to do and both baby and mother receive the benefits. Be careful your feet do not leave the mat when bouncing babies on the rebounder. Because of the increased G-Force at the bottom of the bounce, be sure to support the baby's head and neck carefully. And of course, Don't Drop the Baby!

As the baby continues to grow mother and father should take turns holding the child while rebounding. As the child learns to sit up he/she should be sitting on the rebounder between the feet of mom or dad while they continue their rebound exercise programs. Even before the child begins to walk, he/she will be able to stand on the rebounder and holding on to adult fingers he/she can attempt to get the rebounder to bounce.

When the child is learning to walk I can't think of a better exercise, because rebounding stimulates all of the balancing mechanisms the child will need to put one foot in front of the other.

Parents, you need to make sure your rebounder is readily available in the most enjoyable part of the house, so all your children will rebound practically without thinking. This will help them to become habitual rebounders.

There are four critical years between the time a child begins to walk and the time they start kindergarten. During that time the little body will attempt to get right with the gravitational pull of the earth and the more we can assist their small bodies in achieving that task, the better prepared the child is going to be when he/she is confronted with learning in school. School, now there's a real challenge. But each child somehow gets through it.

Preschool Program

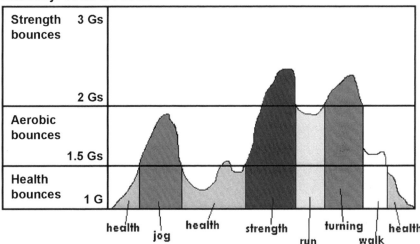

Before kindergarten, children's learning responsibilities are limited to their surrounding environment, communicating with family members and learning of their own anatomy. Formal education begins when kindergarten exposes the child to the world of virtual reality. Before, marks on paper or a television screen meant nothing to the child, now each mark has a value. Lines, curves and colors now represent something created in the complex imagination of the community. Strange marks now have sounds and names. Colors can be divided and subdivided. Single numbers and individual letters have only a name by which each are identified, but combined with other numbers or letters and they mean something new.

At this point, the more solidly a child can comprehend and grasp each nuance of the educational process, the easier it will be to cope with the demands placed upon them. Since all of the cells of this child's body are in the process of learning their individual and collective function, a rebounder is one of the best if not the very best tool for stimulating the educational process at the cell level. At the bottom of the bounce all cells are stimulated individually. The cells react and make the necessary adjustments. Each cell is more adjusted and intelligent about its surrounding environment. This is known as "Rebound Education." It works.

Youth

Youth Beginner

Intensity/ Total G-Force

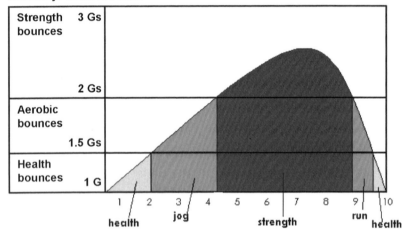

Do you remember your clumsy years? That time in your life when you were all knees, elbows, eyeballs, ears, hands and feet? It was that period of your life, just before, during and after puberty when all of the cells of your body received instructions from the human growth hormones to become larger, to multiply a few more times and to produce an abundance of protein molecules. These protein molecules in turn became thousands of different enzymes, which caused your body to grow in an organized, though seemingly chaotic way. You remember that time don't you? You were in the fifth, sixth and seventh grades. Remember when the girls were 25% bigger than the boys? Zits on the faces seemed to create a deeper uncontrollable voice in the boys while making the girls blossom into young women. Ah, so you do remember. I believe it is a time we would all like to forget, but all youth have to stumble through it.

The clumsiness happens because all of the cells of the body have conveniently adjusted to a particular body size. Suddenly there is a growth spurt. The arms and legs are no longer in proportion with each other. They are now just long enough to cause the teenagers to stumble, when walking or climbing stairs. This lack of coordination is embarrassing, confusing and sometimes even dangerous.

Youth Goal Program

Intensity/ Total G-Force

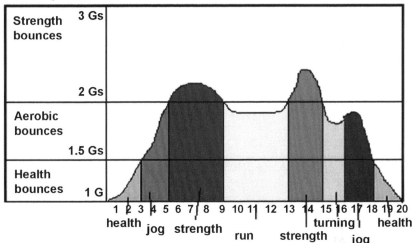

Rebounding during this crucial time is more than just a great idea, it becomes a safety net for saving face among peers. Rebounding will provide strength and aerobic benefits. The primary purposes for youth to rebound is for balance, coordination, rhythm, timing, dexterity and kinesthetic awareness. If our youth rebound daily perhaps they won't have to look back on "those clumsy years" because there will have been less clumsiness.

Teenagers

Let us consider the teenage years as those right after the clumsy years and up until adulthood. It is that period of time when the guys shave once every two weeks, whether they need to or not, and the girls wear blush even when they do not have to. The boys are beginning to think about muscular development and the girls are concentrating on curves. Or perhaps it is the other way around. I do not remember, it was so long ago.

Teenager Goal Program

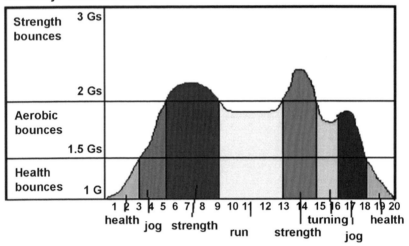

Intensity/ Total G-Force

I remember my son coming home from high school and mentioning that his fellow classmates asked him how he got his six-pack. His friends were surprised when he told them he did not lift weights. He rebounded daily. They had a hard time believing rebound exercise would provide the desired results until his friends began to rebound for themselves and got the same results.

Today there are more obese high school boys and girls than ever before because of their sedentary lifestyle and the availability of convenient fast foods. This obesity does not have to be. Convince a teenage girl to rebound daily for just two weeks and you will probably never have to speak of the benefits of rebounding again. She will see the difference and so will her friends.

Adults

"That looks like a great toy for kids but I do not think I would ever use it."

"How can any thing that simple be so good for you?"

These are responses we get from people who are exposed to re-bound exercise for the first time. There is no doubt rebounding is a great activity for children and a rebounder is a lot of fun to bounce on,

Adult Beginner

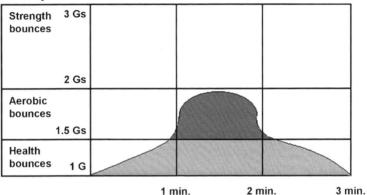

Adult Intermediate

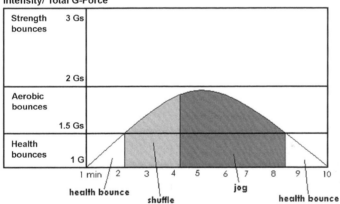

Adult Goal

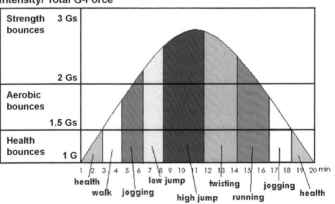

but the people who usually need rebound exercise more than anybody else are the adults. They are the ones who need exercise and they are usually the ones who do not have time for an organized exercise program. They are busy with home, family and professional responsibilities. Many adults have been in such good shape for the first 20 years of their life they have not had to worry about body tone, weight loss or aerobic activities. When they begin to comprehend they need an organized exercise program, most adults do not know where to begin. When they do finally begin, many of them start their exercise program wrong. Here are some suggestions to help you get the best results out of your rebound exercise program. Try these sample workouts or use them to design your own.

The Executive

Daily, I meet many business people who are woefully out of shape and overweight. Some of these business people brag about their physical capability on the football fields, basketball courts, baseball diamonds or tennis courts. Many would tell you of their gymnastic competition in high school and college. They used to be good athletes in excellent condition. Now they are business people who because of their profession sit around all day long in front of a computer or in board meetings making executive decisions. They have read the same statistics you and I have read about how exercise will improve one's efficiency in the workplace. However, work in the daytime does not allow them the privilege of exercising. By the time they commute home, they are too tired to even think about it. For these people, we have developed a rebound exercise program to solve the executive dilemma.

Rebounding and the Executive

Most executives regardless of their athletic background do not have the time to compete in athletic activities. Most really don't have the desire to see how strong they can become or how far they can run. They have the desire to be the best executive they can be so they can secure the greatest financial position for themselves and their families. For these executives we have developed:

Executive Home Program

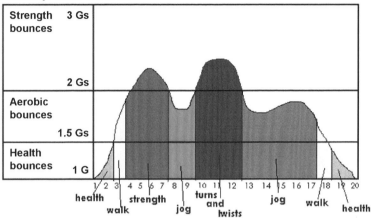

Intensity/ Total G-Force

Strength bounces	3 Gs
Aerobic bounces	2 Gs / 1.5 Gs
Health bounces	1 G

health   walk   strength   jog   turns and twists   jog   walk   health

Executive Office Program

Intensity/ Total G-Force

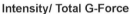

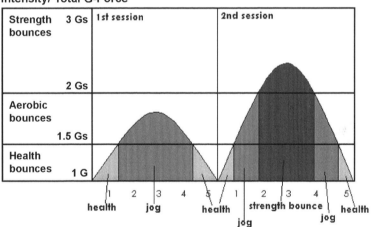

1st session   2nd session

health   jog   health   jog   strength bounce   jog   health

Five Step 3½ Minute
Executive Rebound Fitness Program

Step 1

Begin by rebounding the Health Bounce for thirty seconds. This is a comfortable, stimulating warm-up. It stimulates the lymphatic system and increases metabolism.

Step 2

Continue with the Strength Bounce for one minute. Try to go as high as is comfortable for you. This G-Force loading has the effect of strengthening each muscle and bone cell of the body all at once. Though it does not go through a full range of motion, this G-Force stacking is so efficient it can take the place of all strengthening exercises such as push-ups, sit-ups, pull-ups and weightlifting.

Step 3

Rebound Sprint as fast as you can for one minute. Even the best athletes find this challenging. By the end of one minute you should be breathing rapidly. This rapid breathing is an indication you have used up the available oxygen and your body must replace it. It only takes fifty-five seconds of rapid activity to use up all of the stored creatine phosphate and ATP in the cells. The complete depletion of stored ATP will cause the mitochondria to replicate, thus increasing available energy to burn throughout the day.

Step 4

Return to the Health Bounce for one minute. This will activate the Lymphatic System and will suck out the lactic and uric acids that accumulate in the muscles (anytime one is involved in an aggressive physical activity lactic and uric acids build up in the muscles).

Step 5

Repeat the entire exercise program twice a day. The best time is first thing in the morning and right after you get home from work while you are changing your clothes. If you will carry out this seven-minute exercise program, you will notice a dramatic increase in your productivity throughout the day. Within one week you will notice a strength increase, and more energy to burn—literally.

Pregnancy

It happens to most women more than once. Most of the time the end results are worth the waiting, worrying, wondering, wishing and extra weight. From the time of conception a nine-month clock is ticking. Efficient circulation of body fluids is essential. So, consistent lymphatic stimulation is vitally important to both mother and baby. Mother has a limited amount of time to prepare for the greatest physical demand of her life. The stronger she is, especially during the ninth month of her pregnancy, the healthier and safer it is for both her body and the baby's body. Hormones, enzymes and chemical reactions are going to make sure the body of the baby has everything it needs. Sometimes this process robs vital minerals and vitamins from the skeletal system of the mother. It is important to participate in any ongoing exercise program to reduce the possibility of osteoporosis in later years. The health bounce for body fluid circulation and the aerobic bounce for supplying plenty of oxygen are vitally important during this nine-month period. The aerobic bounces also put a demand on the bones to mineralize.

Rebound exercise is a cellular exercise, providing stimulation for all cells in the body. This includes the placenta and of course the baby. As the baby's vestibular system is developing, rebounding provides pre-birth balancing signals so the child will have a keener sense of balance and a substantial head start.

Baby Boomers

As the generation that was conceived right after the Second World War begins to feel the effects of growing older, many are beginning to look for ways to extend their middle-age and reduce or possibly even eliminate symptoms of old age. Exercise can help to eliminate many of these symptoms, but some people are finding exercise can be hazardous to your health. Before you give up on exercise, you owe it to yourself to get involved with a daily consistent rebound exercise regiment.

Senior Goal

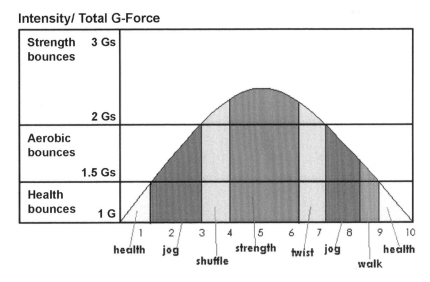

Senior Beginner

Intensity/ Total G-Force

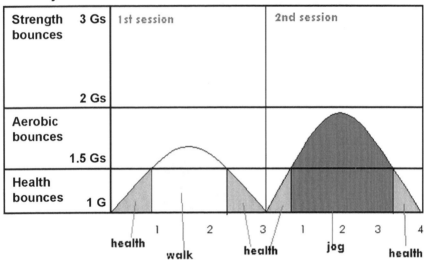

Weight Training and Rebound Exercise

I received a telephone call from Dr. R. Donald Hagan, Ph.D., director of exercise physiology, telling me some of the stories in *The Miracles of Rebound Exercise* were simply too hard to believe. When I told him they were all true, he asked me.

"Are they backed by scientific studies?"

"I am not a scientist." I said. "I am merely reporting what I am learning."

"Well, we need scientific evidence before we can accept rebound exercise as a viable form of exercise."

"You are a scientist aren't you?" I countered. "Why don't you study rebound exercise and report back to me? Besides, it will be more credible if you perform the study rather than if we perform it."

I received a letter confirming our conversation in which he stated they were preparing a research proposal to study rebound exercise. What could be greater than to have Dr. Kenneth Cooper's Institute of Aerobics Research Study conduct the first scientific study of rebound exercise?

The report of the completed study came across my desk six months later. They must have been impressed because this is the way it started out:

The Institute of Aerobics Research Study

NEW

SUPER CIRCUIT PROGRAM

conditions the whole body for

endurance, strength and flexibility.

"These findings will have a significant impact at every level of physical conditioning, whether in high school, college, professional teams, sports medicine or fitness programs."

"The Super Circuit will help move participants through their conditioning program faster with greater overall conditioning effectiveness. And, it will provide much of the needed aerobic conditioning for their particular sport without subjecting their bodies to lifting very heavy weights or jogging great distances in a running program."

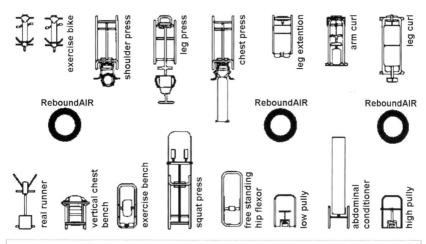

The Institute of Aerobics Research did a study showing that the super circuit produced as much as 25% improvement in strength gains over regular circuit weight training.

This was the fifth study Dr. Larry Gettman, Ph.D., Paul Ward, Ph.D. and R. D. Hagan Ph.D. had undertaken to examine the cardio respiratory aspects of isokinetic and isotonic weight training. It lasted 12 weeks and consisted of 36 females and 41 males who reflected the average condition of normally active people. The only difference between the Super Circuit group and the Regular Circuit weight training control group was those who participated in the Super Circuit rebounded for 30 seconds in between each of the circuit weight training stations.

"These Super Circuit aerobic results are the highest ever reported in literature on circuit weight training—a 17% improvement [in overall fitness over the 12 week period] while the regular Circuit Weight Training groups improved by 12.5%...

"But the Super Circuit has other advantages too. There is less skeletal shock and joint stress..., plus, strength gains showed a 25% improvement over the standard circuit weight training! Plus a Super Circuit develops strength, flexibility and whole body conditioning."

The scientists compared a 30-minute Super Circuit Weight Training program to a regular Circuit Weight Training and 11 other, athletic and recreational sport and daily activities.

"Of these, Super Circuit Weight Training is the only activity capable of conditioning the whole body, providing more aerobic benefits than an hour and a half of rigorous tennis singles or an equivalent of 45 minutes of basketball, plus significantly increasing strength, endurance, flexibility and body fat reduction."

Just to make sure you know what we are talking about, Dr. Larry Gettman's research team simply put rebounders on the same floor with all other circuit weight training devices. He then required all participants in the Super Circuit Weight Training portion of his study to rebound in between each visit to other weight training stations.

The results of this study are certainly fantastic, but it begs the question, can rebound exercise eliminate the need for all other exercise equipment? The answer to that question will astound you.

As mentioned, muscle movement or contraction, is a cellular function. The musculature of the human body is made of communities of cells banded together to perform a task that an individual cell cannot perform by itself, namely, to move a part of the skeletal system. The body is made up of more than 620 of these highly organized communities of muscle cells.

These muscles are able to communicate with each other through a sophisticated, intricate system of neurons, or nerve cells, without which muscle cells are unable to move. Coordination is the combination of the exact message delivered to precise muscle cells at exactly the right moment. For example, the seemingly simple activity of pitching a baseball is a highly complicated movement involving every part of the musculoskeletal system. This includes the large bones, muscles and joints in the legs; large and small bones, muscles and joints of the back; bones, muscles, and joints through the shoulders, arms, wrists, hands and even bones and muscles in the fingertips.

The baseball pitcher thinks nothing of the internal activity of his miraculous body as he winds up to pitch. His thoughts are on the man on first and third, the batter and the message he receives from the catcher. He doesn't have to think of the internal activities of his body because this miraculous machine performs its millions of tasks automatically (once they are learned).

The teachers who help developed these skills in the world's greatest athletes are the very same instructors who teach newborn infants who are just learning the art of grasping mother's little finger. They are the very same teachers who taught our space scientists how to calculate the trajectory of an inbound space capsule bearing our astronauts. And those teachers are none other than the ever present, never changing downward pull of gravity and the two ever changing G-Forces of movement—acceleration and deceleration. Every movement of man or beast is a combination of reactions to one or more of these three forces. Our athletes are those who have been able to learn from these three masters.

Rebound exercise uniquely combines these three forces (or teachers). Only with rebound exercise are they stacked together in a vertical direction. This neuromuscular phenomenon can be found nowhere else in this world. Although it is unique, the serious athlete has left it largely un-investigated, until now.

Dr. Sneider Improves on the Most Efficient Form of Exercise

"I know how to make rebound exercise even better," I heard one day when I was at the National Health Federation convention in Anaheim, California. The voice belonged to Dr. Harry Sneider, fitness coach of Ambassador College in Pasadena, California.

"If you can improve upon the rebound exercise, you have my undivided attention," I said. That was the beginning of Aerobic Resistive Rebounding, a simple concept of putting 1, 2 or 3 pound lightweights in the hands and running, jumping or bouncing on a rebounder while moving the weights in the hands in organized motions.

Harry Sneider, Ph.D. "Dr. Fit" is a world renowned authority in fitness education, Olympic coaching and a world champion weightlifter. His wife,

Sarah Sneider, B.A. is a nutrition and human development graduate and is certified by the American Council on Exercise. She teaches exercise, dance and does fitness testing. They are the owners and creators of the very innovative system, Aerobic Resistive Rebounding, and have been teaching rebound classes for over 40 years combined. Thousands of students follow their fitness program worldwide.

Harry and Sarah Sneider, authors of the book *Olympic Trainer,* have combined the universally-accepted exercise concept of resistance with the revolutionary new cellular exercise concept of rebounding. This new system not only assists in building muscle, bulk and strength but also teaches the body the necessary skills of balance, coordination, rhythm, timing, dexterity and kinesthetic awareness. Aerobic Resistive Rebounding also provides a refreshing aerobic activity void of the joint jarring shock of hitting a hard surface.

"I feel this imaginative system of exercises will revolutionize the exercise methods of our world-class athletes," claims Sneider. It is a system Harry has already proven successful with some of our best athletes, but it can and should be used by everyone from the weakest to the strongest, from the clumsiest to the most fleet of foot. Do not be fooled by its simplicity. Prove it to yourself for yourself.

You can throw away the Universal Gyms, the treadmills and almost any other exercise equipment you have been using in the past. A good rebound unit, your weights and your logbook are all you need for a super bodybuilding fitness program.

Do not go cheap on your rebounder. The inexpensive mini-trampolines you may find at local sporting goods stores, departament stores or superstores are little more than toys. The springs are small, brittle and break easily. The fabric of the mat is questionable. The legs screw on which means they can be screwed off and lost. Our quality, resilient, well built rebounders come with a lifetime warranty. So, do not settle for anything but the very best.

Most people have a tendency to go after the 5 and 10 pound weights because that is what they're used to using in health clubs. Except for the all ready well built athlete 5 and 10 pound weights are too heavy to effectively carry on any resistive rebound programs. We have found 1, 2 or 3 pound weights are adequate for a rebound exercise program. The combined forces of gravity and acceleration can make hand weights about 2–3 times their actual weight at the bottom of the bounce. You will also be lifting the weights rapidly, so the smaller weights will suffice.

It is not necessary to spend too much money on weights. Go to your pantry and pull out a couple of cans of soup or fill two baby bottles with water. My preference would be a couple of plastic baby bottles rather than cans of soup. Of course, that might be because I have had the unpleasant experience of dropping a can of soup on my toe while rebounding.

For those of you who would like inexpensive drop-resistant rebound weights, we offer 1 pound and 3 pound palm weights. These weights fit on to the hand, like a glove and are strapped around the wrists with Velcro. The weight is on the palm of your hand (thus, the name palm weights) or you can wear them on the back of your hands, so you can use each hand for other things while you are rebounding.

Your logbook should be a spiral notebook, which you will use to login your daily exercise programs. Set up your logbook, so you can schedule in advance, what you plan to do each time you rebound with your resistance weights. Then record what you actually did do every day. Your logbook is important because it will help you look back to the beginning of your exercise program. You can then be motivated by how far and how fast you are progressing in your weight training bodybuilding activity.

The Olympic Trainer Introduces us to the Daily Dozen

After you warm up with the health bounce, pick up your weights and go through each of the following movements 10 times. Memorize them, so you can go through them in a systematic way. The daily dozen will take just a few minutes. In addition to their specific purposes, each one of these exercises works the entire cardiovascular system.

Curl

Firmly grip your one pound weights, cans of soup or baby bottles filled with water in your hands. Rebound jog or rebound shuffle in the center of the mat, with your palms up and your elbows close to your side. Raise both weights together to your shoulders. Then bring the weights back to their original position.

Purpose: This is a great exercise that builds and firms the biceps, the forearms and the hand grip. It also works the muscles of the legs, the abdomen and the back.

Press

Firmly grip your weights in your hands, jog or shuffle in the center of the mat. Begin with your weights at your shoulders. Extend both weights together vertically overhead and bring them back to your shoulders.

Purpose: This is a wonderful exercise for the upper back, shoulders and arms. It is excellent for overall toning of the arms.

Upright Row

Firmly grip your one pound weights in your hands and jog, shuffle or bounce in the center of the mat. Begin with your arms together extended downward in front of you (palms down). Pull your hands to your chin with your elbows high. Then lower your hands to their original position.

Purpose: This is an excellent exercise for posture, upper back, shoulders, chest and forearms.

Triceps Press

Firmly grip your weights in your hands and jog, shuffle or bounce in the center of the mat. Place your hands behind your head and extend your forearms upward, then bring them back down to their original position behind your head.

Purpose: This exercise concentrates on the triceps (back of the upper arms), shoulders and grip.

Squeeze

Hold your one pound weights in front of your body at shoulder height while you jog shuffle or bounce in the center of the mat. Squeeze firmly for eight seconds and release.

Purpose: This is a great exercise for the biceps triceps for arms and your grip.

Curl & Press

Firmly grip your one pound weights in your hands and jog, shuffle or bounce in the center of the mat. With your palms up and elbows to your side, pull your weights to your shoulders. From the shoulder position, push both weights vertically overhead. Then bring your weights back to your shoulders and then back to the original position.

Purpose: This is excellent for shaping the arms (front and back), the upper chest and the forearms.

Side Raise

Firmly grip your weights and jog, shuffle or bounce in the center of the mat. Holding your arms straight, raise your weights on each side to at least shoulder level without bending your elbows. Then lower them back down to your sides again.

Purpose: This works the shoulders (deltoids), arms and upper back.

Crossovers

Firmly grip the weights while you jog, shuffle or bounce in the center of the mat. Raise your weights out to your sides at shoulder level. Keeping your arms at shoulder level, bend your elbows slightly and cross your arms in front of you with the right arm slightly above the left arm. The next time cross your arms in front of you with the left arm slightly above the right arm.

Purpose: this exercise firms the upper chest, shapes the arms in shoulders and strengthens the upper back.

Sprint Knee High

Grip your one pound weights and begin running in place with your knees waist high. Bring your left arm forward as your right knee comes up and bring your right arm forward as your left knee comes up. Continue this vigorous activity for 15 seconds.

Purpose: This is excellent conditioning for all muscles of the body, specifically waist, hips, thighs, calves and upper body.

Press Up & Out

Firmly grip your one pound weights in your hands and jog, shuffle or bounce in the center of the mat. Begin with your weights at your shoulders and push them vertically overhead. Then bring them back to the shoulders. Now push the weights out to the sides. Then bring them back to the shoulders. Alternate by pressing overhead and then pressing to the sides.

Purpose: This firms the upper back, shoulders, arms and chest.

Pullover

Firmly grip your weights in your hands and jog, shuffle or bounce in the center of the mat. Start with both weights together in front of your body. Then with an arcing movement pull them over your head touching the back of your head. Then bring them back to their original position in front of you.

Purpose: This is an excellent shaping exercise for the chest, shoulders, arms and even waist.

Jog Easy

Firmly grip your one pound weights in your hands and jog easy in the center of the mat. Your elbows and knees should be moving opposite each other in an easy cadence.

Purpose: This is an overall good body conditioner.

You can get a greater understanding of the Daily Dozen by purchasing your copy of Harry and Sarah Sneider's *Olympic Trainer* from Sneider's Family Fitness, Inc., 115 Loralyn Dr., Arcadia, CA 91006.

As soon as you have memorized the daily dozen routine there are several ways you can enhance or increase the resistance of the exercise.

- Increase the weights in your hands from 1 lb. to 3 lbs.
- Increase the number of repetitions from 10 to 12 or 15.
- Increase the number of sets from 1 to 2 or 3.
- Increase the intensity of the jogging activity.
- Increase the altitude of the strength bounce.
- Increase the overall time for the exercise from 15 minutes to 20 or 30.
- Consider using any of the above in combination.

Let's take a closer look at Aerobic Resistive Rebounding

A close analysis of the concept of hand held weights while rebounding will reveal remarkable results. If one stands on the rebounder and holds a one pound weight in each hand, it will exert an extra one pound of weight on each arm, a total of 2 pounds on the trunk and legs. This can be verified by standing on a bathroom scale and having someone hand you the two one pound weights.

If one jumps on a rebound unit creating 2Gs of gravitational force, the weight will then be translated by the muscle and bone cells of the body as two extra pounds on each arm at the bottom of the bounce or a total of four pounds on the trunk and legs. If one creates the bounce by rhythmically moving the weights up and down, the G-Force is at least doubled again at the bottom of the bounce and 1G of deceleration at the top of the bounce. The cells of the arms translate this into the work of five pounds of resistance for each arm or a total of ten pounds for the trunk and legs. If you move the weights one foot while you are sinking into the mat six inches and bouncing six inches, the weights have been moved a total of ten feet for each bounce. Assume you bounced six inches off the mat a hundred times a minute, moving the weights one foot using a curl exercise, it would be like moving ten pounds X two feet X one hundred bounces or two thousand foot/pounds in one minute.

10 lbs. X 2ft. X 100 bounces = 2000 ft./1b.

If you used two pound weights, it would be four thousand foot/pounds or if you used three pound weights, it would be six thousand foot/pounds.

For the purpose of illustration, let's assume you use the two pound weights moving them an average of one foot while bouncing six inches off the mat and sinking six inches into the mat. Let's say, you complete the Daily Dozen in Harry and Sarah Sneider's *Olympic Trainer*, twenty-five repetitions, three sets. It takes you twenty minutes. This would be the equivalent of moving a forty ton freight car one foot in twenty minutes, a Volkswagen up forty steps in twenty minutes or curling a one hundred pound barbell two hundred times in twenty minutes!

That is just from moving the weight in your hands! What about your body? Assume you weigh one hundred-fifty pounds and are bouncing high enough to create 2Gs. At the bottom of the bounce you would weigh three hundred pounds. Your entire weight is moved one foot vertically one hundred times each minute, times twenty minutes! That would be the equivalent of moving a three hundred ton freight train engine one foot in twenty minutes! Add that to the forty ton freight car and you will begin to understand why rebound exercise and hand held weights are destined to revolutionize the world's concept of weight training.

You can purchase your own ReboundAIR rebounder at
www.ReboundAIR.com or call in at 1(888) 464-5867(JUMP).

Appendix

Here's How Others are Benefitting from Rebound Exercise

Dear Mr. Carter,

My name is Dr. Larry Helveston. I practice in a small town called Lake City, Tennessee. My wife and I, who is also a naturopathic doctor, practice chiropractic and nutritional counseling and consulting. A few months back I myself got into serious health trouble. I was having gall bladder attacks that were referring pain to my upper back and chest area. I was concerned that I might be having a heart attack. I went to the local medical doctor and had an EKG run just to be sure. It showed nothing but he did find my blood pressure to be dangerously high, (171/102) and wanted me to go on medication to bring it under control. Boy, did that ever wake me up, here I was teaching others how to be healthy and me in this kind of trouble!! Well that did it for me, I decided right then that I was not going to succumb to degenerative disease and accept what the medical doctor told me, that it was just part of growing older. (I'm 53)

Four months ago I was approximately 220 lbs, 5'8" tall, out of shape and certainly not fit. I had just read or heard on a tape from a nutrition-ist that the quickest physical way he knew of to lower blood pressure was rebounding. The next thing I knew I was researching your web site study-ing about rebounding. I said, what have I got to loose. I ordered my first rebounder about four months ago and have been hooked ever since. I'm now approaching 170 lbs, my blood pressure averages 124/64, I have more energy than I know what to do with. I just plain ol' feel great!! We have also changed our diet greatly and eat healthy and drink over 100 oz. of distilled water a day. I'm also using your meal matrix to feed me cellularlly.

When I first started rebounding I could hardly do 5 minutes at a time, I was that out of shape!! Now I'm up to 45 minutes per day of resistive rebounding with wrist and ankle weights. We do what we call disco dance rebounding and jump to the beat of the music. It is really fun and doesn't feel like exercise at all!! I rebound seven days a week. I also do strength training 3 days a week on a total gym. I can't say enough about your product and what it has done for me and my family!! We now have two in our office and we recommend them to all our patients...Even my sweet 74 yr. old mother has ordered one and she can't wait to get it!

Sincerely,
Drs. Larry and Teresa Helveston

Hello Again,

Thank you for our pleasant conversation yesterday. I just wanted to take a moment to reiterate some of the reasons I'm truly enjoying the rebounder your company makes. As I mentioned, my wife purchased a ReboundAIR through Ariel Moss, a personal friend of ours for many years, after her enthusiastic recommendation.

When it arrived, I liked the construction of it, and knew it was a serious piece of exercise equipment that was well designed. I read the book my wife also received (The New Miracles of Rebound Exercise) and was quite impressed with the data presented by Mr. Carter. After watching the video (Keep on Rebounding), I was hooked. That was 3 months ago; now my wife can't get me off the thing!

As a physician, I'm aware of the problems of degenerative diseases and the new information attempting to help us all achieve healthy aging. Diet, exercise, and nutritional supplementation seem to be an important part of this equation.

What I like most about the rebounder is it's regular use can help maintain muscle mass, bone density, aerobic capacity, balance, cardiovascular fitness, and reduce insulin resistance—all of which become problematic as we age.

Additionally, it's easy and pleasurable to use, has no parts to essentially break down, is portable, and most important of all, quiet (I have to exercise very early in the morning before work, and I can use the rebounder easily without waking the whole house.) It's the first type of exercise that I've been able to do consistently every day as part of my overall health routine. Since beginning, I've noticed improved stamina, overall strength, balance, flexibility, decreased stress, and better sleep—all without stress on my joints. I have even knocked several strokes off my golf game!

I have owned a NordicTrack, and a treadmill, done cycling, swimming, and jogging, and used gym equipment; this far exceeds the benefits I received from those types of exercise.

Adding a light weight routine a few days a week while jogging on the rebounder rounds out a perfect regimen for me that only takes me about 25 minutes daily. I'm truly delighted with the quality and design of the rebounder, and I appreciate all of the research and time your company has put into producing such a quality exercise aid.

Thank you.
Sincerely—Martin Towbin, M.D.

Hi Al!

I have been looking at your website, and thought I'd share my experience so far. I bought your book many years ago, and a rebounder. I remembered being stronger, faster, and more enthusiastic than almost everyone I knew when I was young. (Teens). I didn't correlate it with the fact that my favorite activity was bouncing on a friends trampoline, which we did (me and my two friends) taking turns for maybe three hours virtually every day. As a young adult I ran everywhere just because I loved moving fast, being athletic, and I felt so good. I was wearing 30/30 size pants throughout most of my twenties, and ate everything I could possibly eat.

Well, at about 26, I had gotten far from regular physical activity, and my diet was poor. I began to gain weight rapidly. By my mid thirties, I had a fairly serious weight problem...

When I was looking at various kinds of exercise equipment, and realized there was nothing I would like more than, or that would provide the health benefits of rebounding. (I must have read your book 'The

New Miracle of Rebound Exercise' at least a half dozen times) By then I had found an old used NordicTrack ski trainer at a rummage sale, and was beginning to use that to get in shape. I did find, however, that I was having some back pain after I used the NordicTrack. I had tried Gym memberships a couple different times, and always wound up getting hurt and dropping out.

Because I had just come into some cash, and placed a high priority on getting into better shape, I had budgeted for some gym equipment for my home. It dawned on me that for the price of a home gym I could get both a good quality full sized trampoline, and a couple rebounders, which I ordered.

I was in for kind of a shock, though. At almost three hundred pounds I had grown too inflexible to bend at the waist sufficiently to do a seat drop so, I couldn't do but very few of the gymnastic things I used to as a teenager on my friends' trampoline. Again feeling kind of discouraged, I didn't take full advantage of my new equipment.

The bright spot was your excellent customer service. I got two quarter-fold rebounders, and one of them broke a clevis pin almost the first week. I called customer service, and without any cost to me they sent me a replacement rebounder within less than a week. I boxed the one with the faulty clevis pin and sent it back in the same box at zero cost to me. ...yup, that one faulty clevis pin... that was me! (Robin is referring to the one and only clevis pin ever recorded to have broken, see Lifetime Warranty Progress Report at www.healthbounce.com/warranty.htm for more information.)

So, what happened when I finally started using the rebounder regularly? Well, I started dieting about a month and a half ago, and using the rebounder daily about the same time for about five minutes twice daily. I also started regular stretching nightly before going to sleep.

Now I find I've lost about thirty pounds (total... about twenty-five since then), but I'm recovering the flexibility I had as a kid. I ran some the last two days. I haven't run at all for about five years until now. My energy level is soaring, and I'm doing more rebounding just because it feels so good and is so FUN!

I recently re-read the book, and have been telling people about the benefits of rebounding, and just got a check for selling someone a rebounder, because I also am a distributor (since I wanted to buy my second rebounder wholesale and the kit was only fifty bucks). All I did was talk about all I had learned from you, and send them to your website.

Anyway, I guess I'm trying to say THANKS for changing my life in so many positive ways!

So, Thanks a million!

Robin Boone, North Carolina

Al Carter,

I purchased my ReboundAIR about a year ago and have been so pleased with it. I bought the ReboundAIR because I was impressed by the lifetime warranty and the construction. After a year my ReboundAIR still looks and feels like new.

Prior to buying my ReboundAIR I had walked mainly for exercise, but I found that my ankles were starting to hurt and I was having lower back pain. I have not had any ankle or back pain since using the ReboundAIR. I started using it about 3 times per week, but for the last couple of months I've increased my workouts to about 4 or 5 times per week and now I'm really seeing some of my old flab and weight I couldn't lose drop off. I look forward to my rebound workouts and even when I feel tired I find that 5 or 10 minutes of simple bouncing helps restore my energy.

By the way, I originally bought all the videos and DVDs that you have on your website. They're great and still challenge me...

Thanks so, much!

Michelle Sandoval Ouray, CO

Hi Al

I started rebounding 28 days ago! My immune system was so,shot and I was tired of being tired and sick. I started with the gentle "health bounce" for 15 min in the morning and 15 min in the evening. I also began a sensible diet to help cut down food allergies etc. My main objective is to get my lymphatic system moving and find some type of exercise I could do without re-injuring my knee (I had the ACL replaced back in '93 and I tore the cartilage off the bone so, no more running or much of anything without severe pain and bleeding in the joint!) so, needless to say, I have been desperate to find an exercise I could do that wouldn't irritate the bones in my knee.

I began to lose weight immediately! Muscle tone, improved breathing, no more ear aches or sore throats and my allergies are clearing up!!!!!

WOW!

I'm up to 38 min in the am and I do about 15 at night. I decided to look up rebounding on the web to find out more about it–need I say more? I found the ReboundAIR and ordered the book and a video for myself and one for my children.

I've been using the "Keep on Rebounding" video for about 2 weeks. I have lost a total of 15 lbs. since I started. I'm toned, slim, my skin is clear and glowing. I still haven't gotten all the moves down in the video, but my knee has strengthened enough to keep my balance and I can at least keep going to the end. My mom started about a week ago and my HUSBAND started about 3 days ago.

I haven't had any pain, I love the results and I'm thinking about getting certified in reboundology and putting an ad in my children's school handout to teach anyone else who wants to learn. It's amazing. I am very excited about this and I love my Quarter Fold ReboundAIR, it's so much nicer than the one I picked up at a 2nd hand sports place. Even less impact on my knee and joints. I could add a list of things that have improved, but I figure this is long enough.

Thanks for a great product and for a great video!

Stephanie Jemmett

Hello Al:

My name is Ray Koncsol. I'm a 62 year old gentleman that was diagnosed as having Muscular Dystrophy in 1976 in Pittsburgh, PA. In 1981 I retired in Florida and weighed about 225 lbs. In 1983 I bought the book "The Miracles of Rebounding" and my first rebounder. I have kept your book at my bedside for many years and have read it so much that I have had to use tape to keep it bound together.

Over the years my rebounding has gone from 45 minutes a day to nothing. Sometimes when I got really lazy and would not rebound for a long time, my mobility would get so bad that I could hardly walk without looking like I'm going to fall over any minute.

Other times when I was on a streak of consistent daily exercise I would walk so normal that when I would tell people that I had MD they would say they hadn't noticed anything in my walking.

What I'm trying to say is that I have to sincerely say that I believe that rebound exercise has kept me out of a wheelchair for the last 18 years or at least the last 5 years. I have a record of every jump I've ever done on a rebounder kept in annual diaries and I can look back and tell the good years from the bad years according to how much time I spent on the re-bounder.

I have to put my rebounder in the hallway and hold onto the door jambs because my balance is not so good but right now I'm back to re-bounding almost daily (I've rebounded 93 out of the last 96 days). I have atrophy in the front of my ankles so, even when I'm doing the strength bounce my toes will not leave the mat but I do the best that I can.

Over the last 3 months, I've sometimes rebounded for 30 minutes a day and sometimes for over 50 minutes a day. I've made a promise to myself that I'm going to do at least something every day no matter what.

I now weigh about 185 lbs and would like to lose about 20 lbs in the midsection and have that as my goal over the next year. My main goal through rebounding to make myself a productive person as far as income is concerned so, I'm not a burden to my son or my family. I would like to become a member of your organization but will have to wait until I can get the funds together to get one of your units. I came across your web-site last week and have spent hours looking at everything I could find on rebounding.

It's really nice to see how rebounding may finally get the recognition that it certainly deserves. I hope I can be a part of introducing the best exercise known to man to a truly uneducated public. I wanted to write and thank you for what you introduced back in 1979 because as I said be-fore.......I would be in a wheelchair if I had not read your book and started rebounding.

Thanks a Million ! ! !
Ray Koncsol

Dear Sirs:

Just a note to tell you about the results with my rebounder. I'm now 54 years old, and 4 years ago I purchased a rebounder from you. Prior to using the rebounder, I had experienced headaches for 10 years or more. These headaches occurred anywhere from 3 to 15 days apart, and would last up to 30 hours, during which time it was difficult for me to work or think effectively. The headaches grew more severe over the years, and also more frequent.

When I first began to use the rebounder, my head would throb somewhat if I tilted it front, back or sideways as I bounced, and I noticed that mucus was draining from the sinus cavities in my head down into my throat. As I used the rebounder for 15–20 minutes a day for about 6 months, my headaches decreased in both frequency and intensity, to only about 20% of their previous levels. They have remained at these lower levels with continued use of the rebounder.

Another benefit I experienced with rebounding had to do with my voice. I have been involved with church music all of my adult life, and began to notice around 1997 that my singing voice was growing weaker, for no apparent reason. I could not sing with much power, particularly in the upper register. The rebounding did something in my larynx and throat which restored my singing voice beautifully. I am very thankful to the Lord for this. I find that keeping up with the rebounding helps maintain my headache-reduced and voice-improved condition. Thank you for your product.

Sincerely,

Ed Myers
Kansas

Glossary of Terms

Acceleration—Expression of the rate of change in velocity. Increase in rapidity of motion or function.

Aerobic exercise—Oxygen utilization activities characterized by moderate intensities, long duration and large muscle group or "whole body" repetitive movements. The primary fuel for aerobic metabolism is fat ($CH_3(CH_2)14COOH$) and carbohydrates ($C_6H_{12}O_6$). The by-products of aerobic metabolism are water (H_2O), carbon dioxide (Co_2) and heat.

Aerobic Resistive Rebounding—Aerobic exercises on a rebounder while utilizing hand held weights. Rebounding increases the G-Force applied to the weights, which in turn benefits the entire body.

Anaerobic exercise—Activity during which the energy needed is provided without utilization of oxygen. These types of exercise are characterized by short burst, higher intensity movements such as weight lifting and sprinting. An aerobic routine can quickly become anaerobic if a level of intensity is reached at which the body is not accustomed. The fuel for anaerobic metabolism is glycogen and the by-products are lactic acid and heat.

Angina—(angina pectoris) Severe pain and a sensation of constriction around the heart. The condition is caused by a restriction of oxygen to a segment of the heart muscle (myocardium). Typically, pain radiates to the left arm and shoulder. Sometimes the pain is also felt in the back and jaw. Rarely, angina radiates to the abdomen.

Antibodies—Specially shaped proteins produced by the body's army of white blood cells which neutralize or destroy foreign proteins (antigens). When infected with virus or bacteria, the body produces antibodies that destroy the invading microorganisms.

Arteriosclerosis—Hardening of the layers of the arterial walls. Associated with high blood cholesterol and lipid levels, smoking, obesity, hypertension, sedentary lifestyle, heredity, diabetes and inability to cope with stress. Arteriosclerosis is the leading cause of death in the western world. [(1)*Tabor's Cyclopedic Medical Dictionary...*]

ATP-CP—A quick energy release anaerobic compound, fueled by sugar, for short-burst and high intensity activity. The by-product of this chemical reaction is lactic acid and heat.

Basal metabolic rate—Lowest level of energy expenditure at complete rest. For an average person, this is approximately 1500–1800 Calories per day. [Taber's]

Blood pressure—The pressure of the blood in the main arteries which rises and falls as the cardiac and arteriole muscles of the body cope with varying demands (e.g. exercise, stress, sleep). There are two types of pressures that are measured:systolic pressure, created by the contraction of the heart muscle and diastolic pressure, the residual pressure within the arteries when the heart is at rest between beats. Example of a normal blood pressure: 120/80 (systolic over diastolic)

Body composition—Fat to lean body mass comparison. Superior to scales for assessing health and health risks, hydrostatic weighing is an accurate method of measuring body composition.

Bradycardia—A slow heart rate of 60 beats per minute or less.

Cardiac output—Amount of blood pumped from the left or right ventricle chamber per minute. For a male adult at rest, this is approximately 5.6 liters per minute. [(2) Guyton's Textbook of *Medical Physiology*. p.239] Cardiac output is determined by multiplying the stroke volume by the heart rate. (see stroke volume)

Cholesterol—A monohydric alcohol associated with animal fats. Cholesterol is important in the endocrine (hormone) system of the body. The desirable level of cholesterol in the blood is less than 200 mg/dl. [Taber's]

Conditioning—Improving the physical capability by adaptation to a designed stress.

Connective tissue—Tissue that supports, surrounds and protects other tissues and body parts. Examples: bones, skin, muscle, ligaments, tendons, cartilage and fascia. These tissues, by virtue of their position and function, adapt to moderate increases in external forces (such as exercise) by becoming more dense (as in the calcification of bone) or by protein synthesis of fibers that augment strength of the tissue (as in the actin and myosin filaments within muscle cell).

Deceleration—Negative acceleration or decrease in velocity.

DNA—(deoxyribonucleic acid) The "blueprints of the cell". The chemical basis of genetics. The carrier of structure and function information for all organisms. DNA is found within the nucleus of each cell and is arranged in two long chains that twist around each other to form a double helix.

Dyspnea—A hunger for air, accompanied by labored breathing and sometimes pain.

Electrolytes—Minerals that, in a solution, conduct electricity. Common electrolytes in the body are sodium, potassium and chlorine. These are important for the propagation of action potentials across the membranes of neurons. Also, electrolytes are essential for balancing the intracellular and extracellular fluid volumes such as the function of the sodium-potassium pump of the cell membrane. Profuse perspiration, dehydration, vomiting or diarrhea tends to disturb the delicate concentrations of the electrolytes in the body.

Enzyme—A protein complex that stimulates chemical reactions within other substances without being changed itself. "The factory worker inside the cell."

Exercise prescription—A personalized exercise routine specifying type (or mode), frequency, duration and intensity of activity.

Fatigue—A feeling of tiredness or weariness. The condition of a tissue or organ in which its response to stimulation is reduced. Fatigue may be the result of excessive activity, which results in the accumulation of lactic acid. Other causes of fatigue include malnutrition, heart disease, anemia, respiratory disturbances, infection, hormone disturbances such as hyperinsulinism (common to diabetics) and menopause. Psychogenic influences include conflicts, frustration, anxiety, neurosis and boredom. Environmental factors include noise and vibration.

Free fatty acids—Fats (lipids) in mobilized form.

Glucose—Blood sugar; primarily obtained by dietary carbohydrates. The normal range is 80–100mg/dl.

Glycogen—Sugar in storage form within the muscle.

Gravity—The universal attraction of matter to matter. The attraction of the moon to the earth, the earth to the sun, the force that holds us to the surface of the earth.

HDL—(High-density lipoprotein) A chemical compound, formed in the liver, with a high concentration of protein, about 50%, but smaller concentrations of cholesterol and phospholipids. HDL removes excess cholesterol from the bloodstream. A high HDL to LDL ratio reduces the likelihood of developing atherosclerosis. [Guyton's, p. 875] (see also LDL)

Health—A state of potential energy; the ability to carry out all daily activities with mental clarity and physical endurance. A lack of disease.

Heart murmur—Heard through a physician's stethoscope, it is the sound of turbulent blood passing through the heart. Heart murmurs are possible indications of abnormal blood flow and may be caused by a disorder such as narrowing (stenosis) or leaking (regurgitation) of a heart valve (structure which opens to allow blood to flow away from the heart and closes to prevent back flow into the heart). Many murmurs are benign (of no significance).

Hydrostatics—The science of properties of fluids in equilibrium.

Hypertension—High blood pressure, measured above 140/90. If uncontrolled, hypertension could lead to artery, heart, kidney and brain damage.

Hypotension—Low blood pressure, usually blood pressure measured below 90/60.

Hypoxia—Insufficient supply or very low saturation of oxygen in the blood or tissue.

Ischemia—Disturbance of the blood flow to a muscle or tissue. Commonly refers to a deprived segment of the heart muscle due to a narrowing of a coronary artery.

Immune system—The processes and specialized cells used by the body to identify abnormal or foreign bodies and prevent them from harming the organism.

Isometric contraction—Muscle contraction without movement of the limb. No muscle lengthening or shortening occurs. An example is attempting to move an immovable object.

Isotonic contraction—Muscle contraction with movement of the limb. The muscle lengthens or shortens. Example: weight lifting.

Kilogram—(kg) Metric unit of weight equivalent to 2.2 lb.

Krebs cycle—(citric acid cycle) [Named for Sir Hans Krebs, German biochemist, 1900–1981, co-winner of a Nobel prize in 1953.] A complicated cascade of reactions in the mitochondria involving the oxidative metabolism of pyruvic acid and the liberation of energy in the eventual formation of numerous ATP.

Lactic acid—Lactic acid is the probable cause of delayed onset muscle soreness (DOMS). [Taber's] It is formed during muscular activity by the breakdown of glycogen. Lactic acid is produced at a faster rate when there is inadequate oxygenation of skeletal muscle or the demand for contraction exceeds the muscle cells' conditioned capacity to produce ATP within the Krebs cycle of the mitochondria. Over time, exercise will cause more capillaries to form around and near the muscle cells. More mitochondria will be replicated within the muscle cells specifically used for the activity. This increase in mitochondria count will enable the cells to produce an adequate supply of ATP to meet the demands of the activity. With the body now able to utilize oxygen at shorter notice, for longer duration and at higher intensities, less lactic acid will be produced. This is one of the more notable changes that occurs within our bodies as we "get into shape". In essence, more capillaries and more mitochondria translate to more endurance and less soreness!

LDL—(low-density lipoprotein) A chemical compound, formed in the liver, with a low concentration of protein and high concentration of cholesterol. The LDL blood count increases with dietary consumption of saturated fats. The primary function of all lipoproteins is fat transportation within the blood stream.

Lymphatic system—All structures involved in the conveyance of lymph from the tissues to the bloodstream. It includes the lymph capillaries, lacteals, lymph nodes, lymph vessels, one-way valves and main lymph ducts (thoracic and right lymphatic ducts). The lymphatic system provides the battlegrounds upon which the body's immunities are continually on search and destroy missions. (see immune system)

Lysosome—An organelle within the cell that digests substances such as damaged cell structures, ingested food particles and bacteria.

Metabolism—The sum total of all chemical reactions required for body growth, function and transformation of chemical energy of food to mechanical energy or heat. Commonly equated to caloric expenditure.

Mitochondria—Called the "powerhouses of the cell". These intracellular organelles recruit the services of oxidative and nutrient enzymes in the synthesis of the body's energy currency, ATP (adenosine triphosphate). The number of mitochondria in each cell varies from less than a hundred up to several thousand depending on the regular amount of energy required by the cell. For example, progressive aerobic exercise dramatically augments the mitochondria count within the muscle cells.

Muscle tissues—3 types compared:

Cardiac muscle—Involuntary control, moderate speed of contraction, striated, displays characteristics of automaticity and synchronicity to function as a vascular pump, contains one nucleus per cell.

Smooth muscle—Involuntary control, very slow wave-like contraction, no striation, found along digestive tract, contains one nucleus per cell.

Striated muscle— Voluntary control, relatively fast speed of contraction, marked striation (fiber stripes) in appearance, connected to bone for movement, each cell contains multiple nuclei.[Taber's]

Nucleus—The "control center of the cell". A vital cell organelle, containing DNA, which orchestrates cell growth, reproduction, metabolism and transmission of genetic characteristics.

Overload Principle—Application to strength development: "Muscles that function under no load increase little in strength. Muscles that contract at more than 50% maximal force of contraction will develop strength rapidly. Using this principle, experiments on muscle development have shown that six nearly maximal muscle contractions performed in three sets three days a week give approximately optimal increase in muscle strength and without producing chronic muscle fatigue." [Guyton's, p.1064]

Pulse—Rate, rhythm, compressibility and tension of the arteries due to the flow pattern of the blood as a result of each heart beat. Normal pulse rate is about 72 in adult males and 80 in adult females.

Pulse pressure— The difference between systolic and diastolic numbers. Normal values should be between 30 and 50 points at rest. [Taber's] Example: 115/70 blood pressure. 115 - 70 = 45 points

Rebounder—An exercise device similar to a trampoline only much smaller. It is perfect for in home, office or personal outdoor use. For more information on rebounders or to purchase your own, contact ReboundAIR at www.ReboundAIR.com or 1(888) 464-5867(JUMP).

Respiration—Exchange of O_2 (oxygen) and CO_2 (carbon dioxide) within the tissues and lungs.

Ribosome—The "assembly platform of the cell". A cell organelle which functions to receive genetic instructions and translates those into protein synthesis.

RNA—(ribonucleic acid) The chemical blueprint copy of DNA segments that controls the synthesis of proteins. RNA is primarily found within the cytoplasm of all living cells. (see DNA)

Solute—A material dissolved in a liquid.

Stroke volume—The amount of blood the heart pumps in one contraction. Amount varies with age, sex and exercise.

Tonus—Involuntary muscle firmness.

Triglycerides—Chain of fats in storage form. Consisting of three fatty acids and one glycerol molecule. Adipose tissue is primary composed of triglycerides.

Vestibular system—Located primarily in the inner ear, consisting of the semi-circular canals, utricle, saccule, cochlea and vestibulochochlear nerve in cooperation with postural reflex portions of the brain stem. The vestibular system aids in the maintenance of equilibrium by sensing the orientation of the head in space with respect to gravity. When in an upright position, our antigravity muscles continuously receive this information, relayed through the brain, resulting in subtle angular, distance and tone adjustments. The vestibular mechanisms also aid in the stabilization of the eyes when the head is in motion. This explains our ability to focus on a chart while bouncing on a rebounder or read a book while jogging on a treadmill.

VO$_2$ max—The maximum amount of oxygen consumed at the tissue level for every kilogram of body weight during the last minute of maximal exercise. Also referred to as oxygen uptake or maximal oxygen consumption. VO$_2$ max is a parameter used to measure fitness. Units represented in kg/min.

Wellness—Spiritual, emotional, mental, physical and social stability and balance.

Weight management—Long-term behavior modification which combines exercise, diet, realistic goals and regular interpersonal support.

Work—The product of force times distance.

For more information, contact:

www.Rebound-Air.com
Facebook.com/ReboundAir
Toll Free 1-888-464-JUMP

www.GoRebound.com
The Rebound Exercise Documentary